In Memoriam: Andrew G. Du Mez (1885 – 1948)

American pharmacist • educator • editor

Publication subvention from the late Mrs. A. G. Du Mez

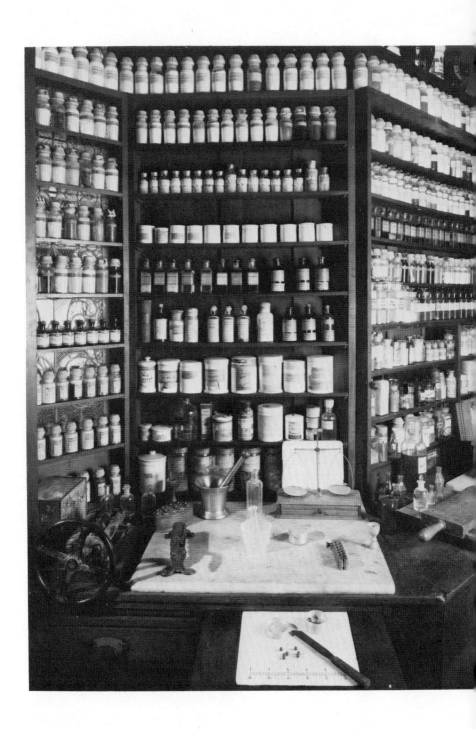

Pharmacy Museums and Historical Collections on Public View in the United States and Canada

Ralaf   19 25 -   alter

SAMI K. HAMARNEH, and **ERNST W. STIEB,** *1929 -*
United States   Canada

American Institute of the History of Pharmacy
Madison, Wisconsin
in cooperation with the
National Museum of American History, Smithsonian Institution
Washington, D.C.
1981

Publication No. 6 (New Series)
John Parascandola, General Editor
American Institute of the History of Pharmacy

Library of Congress Cataloging in Publication Data
Hamarneh, Sami Khalaf, 1925 -
Pharmacy museums and historical collections on public view in
the United States and Canada.
(Publication/American Institute of the History of Pharmacy;
new series, no. 6)
Rev. ed. of: Pharmacy museums and historical collections on
public view, U.S.A.
1. Pharmaceutical museums—United States. 2. Pharmaceutical
museums—Canada—Directories. I. Stieb, Ernst Walter, 1929 -
II. Title. III. Series: Publication (American Institute of the
History of Pharmacy); new series, no. 6.
RS123.U6H35 1981   615'.1'074013   81-2168
ISBN 0-931292-09-3   AACR2

Cover: Laab's apothecary shop is a replica of a Milwaukee,
Wisconsin, store around the turn of the century which contains original period fixtures and shelf ware. (Photo courtesy
of the Milwaukee Public Museum.)

Frontispiece: Detail from a compounding or dispensing area
at the rear of an 1890s' drugstore in the National Museum of
American History (formerly the National Museum of History
and Technology), Smithsonian Institution, Washington, D.C.

Contents

To the American pharmacist—aware of his professional heritage and present achievements, who appreciates the accomplishments that have made American professional pharmacy and the pharmaceutical industry what it is today, and

To those who recognize the aesthetic beauty of the tools, furnishings, and equipment of the past and discover new meanings in them, and who come up with creative ideas in the examination, collection, exhibition, and preservation of pharmaceutical objects, endeavoring to enjoy and appreciate them and to make them the more enjoyable to, and appreciated by, others, and

To all who believe that the future is the offspring of the past and the present and is enriched by their legacy, and therefore are zealous to understand and preserve it,

To such as those, this guidebook of pharmaceutical exhibitions and collections is dedicated.

    S. K. H.

Preface

In the last one hundred years there has been a markedly increased interest in health museums in America, resulting from economic prosperity, increased education and greater cultural awareness, and a developing interest in public health. The Medical Museum of the Armed Forces Institute of Pathology, officially opened in 1862, represented the first-known such institution in North America. Two decades later, in 1881, the Smithsonian Institution established the Section of Materia Medica, then housed at the newly opened Arts and Industries Building. This section eventually developed into the present Division of Medical Sciences at the Smithsonian's National Museum of American History (formerly the National Museum of History and Technology).

Exhibit halls and reference collections of the Division of Medical Sciences now include large sections devoted to pharmaceutical exhibitions and objects and equipment from pharmacy's past. These include, in particular, reconstructions of American and European apothecary shops which display period tools and utensils used in the preparation and manufacture of medications, as well as pharmacy symbols, fixtures and equipment, and portraits and illustrations. From the late 1910s to 1972, except for a short interval, this division was supervised by pharmacist-historians.*

After the turn of this century, prominent individuals in American and Canadian pharmaceutical societies, colleges, and industrial firms, with the aid of funds from private and government sources, fostered the development of several other historical collections, pharmacy museums, and shop restorations. Therefore, a descriptive list of these historical collections became desirable and needed to serve as a guidebook to all those who are interested in these exhibits.

In 1957, under the auspices of the American Institute of the History of Pharmacy, my colleague and predecessor at the Smithsonian Institution, George B. Griffenhagen, prepared a very useful monograph, a brief guide, entitled *American Pharmacy's Historical Collections*. It was

---

*For details, refer to my paper number 43, "History of the Division of Medical Sciences," *United States National Museum Bulletin 240* (Washington, D.C.: Smithsonian Institution, 1964), pp. 269-300.

revised in 1965 by Griffenhagen and Cleo Sonnedecker as a brochure easy to carry on trips. Both publications, as well as Griffenhagen's related booklet, *Tools of the Apothecary* (Washington, D.C., 1957)—a collected series of articles on pharmacy's artifacts—have been out of print for a number of years.

From 1955 to 1956, Griffenhagen authored two other booklets on the same theme: *Early American Pharmacies* (Washington, D.C.: American Pharmacy Association, 1955; 23 pages) and *Pharmacy Museums* (Madison, Wisconsin: American Institute of the History of Pharmacy, 1956; 52 pages). The latter, being an international guide, provided information on major pharmacy museums and collections on public view not only in the United States but elsewhere. It was subsequently incorporated into Glenn Sonnedecker's third and fourth revised editions of *Kremers and Urdang's History of Pharmacy* (Philadelphia: Lippincott, 1963, pages 348-95; and 1976, pages 396-417). Special attention is drawn to this guide because of its wider scope and usefulness. For general references, see also *Museums of the World* (Verlag Dokumentation, Munich: Pullach, 1973), a directory of 17,000 museums in 148 countries with a subject index, and *The Directory of World Museums* (New York: Columbia University Press, 1975) by Kenneth Hudson and Ann Nicholls.

Since the 1965 publication of Griffenhagen and Cleo Sonnedecker's brochure, new collections and pharmacy restorations have appeared, while some others that were open to the public no longer exist. In 1972, therefore, the American Institute of the History of Pharmacy (AIHP) published my *Pharmacy Museums and Historical Collections on Public View, USA*, as an up-to-date guidebook. That work, however, is now out of print. In addition, a number of new museums have opened in the past eight years and other significant changes have also taken place at many of the still-functioning museums that deserve attention. Therefore, it was decided that a revised edition of this guide be made available.

In undertaking the present revision, however, it was also decided that the scope of the work should be expanded to include Canadian museums as well as those in the United States because of the close ties and frequent travel between the two countries. It has been a pleasure and a privilege for me to collaborate with my friend and colleague Ernst W. Stieb, with whom I studied as a fellow graduate student under Glenn Sonnedecker at the University of Wisconsin in the history of pharmacy and science. Dr. Stieb, who is associate dean and professor of the history of pharmacy at the University of Toronto and director of the Canadian Academy of the History of Pharmacy, has taken responsibility for the descriptions of the Canadian museums as well as providing advice and assistance on other portions of this guidebook. Since 1971 he has served as curator of the Niagara Apothecary Museum, where he was responsible for the restoration of the professional practice aspects, and for many years he served as editor of the "Facts about artifacts" and "The past recaptured" columns of *Pharmacy in History*. These useful short descriptive articles have been drawn upon throughout this guide.

In keeping with the scope established for the first edition of this book as well as the previously mentioned two guides, this new edition will be limited to pharmacy museums, apothecary shop restorations, and historical collections on public display. The choice of entries will again exclude strictly private collections maintained by collectors or antique dealers and kept at their homes or places of business, or those which are an integral part of modern operating pharmacies or drug manufacturing companies, or are displayed for decorative purposes in office buildings where visits by the public at large are not encouraged. The scope of this guide also prevents listing of museums and galleries that include within the framework of their larger and main exhibits, pharmaceutical antiques as only a minor part of a more general theme. For information on North American museums in general, the reader should consult the second edition of the *Museum Directory of the United States and Canada* published by the Smithsonian Institution, Washington, D.C., in 1965 and the 1980 edition of *The Official Museum Directory: United States and Canada*, published cooperatively by the American Association of Museums and Macmillian Inc., which provides current and comprehensive information on some 5,225 museums in North America.

Sami K. Hamarneh, curator emeritus, Division of Medical Sciences, Department of the History of Science and Technology, Smithsonian Institution
August 1980

Introduction

To facilitate use, this revised guidebook has been arranged in the
following order. Museums in the United States are described in
alphabetical order by states; also included are the District of Columbia
and Puerto Rico. These are followed by descriptions of Canadian
museums in alphabetical order by provinces presented by coauthor Ernst
Stieb. Both parts are followed by concluding remarks and a listing of
partly annotated published sources of the literature arranged by author
within subject-matter categories. Admission fees are mentioned only
where applicable; otherwise admission is free according to our
information. Fees as well as open hours are, of course, subject to
change. It is advisable to check on such matters, if possible, with the
museum or appropriate local agencies prior to the visit or by making a
special appointment.

It should be noted that in accordance with American custom and
usage, the terms apothecary shop, pharmacy, and drugstore are used
synonymously as they relate to the exhibitions described in the following
entries. We hope that this publication fills a gap in the pharmaceutical
literature. Size and format were restricted to keep it handy as a pocket
companion for the traveler and as a reference for others who, as the
honorary director of the American Institute of the History of Pharmacy,
Glenn Sonnedecker, has written, "would find diversion or instruction in
tangible remains of pharmacy's past."

Professor Sonnedecker, in his foreword to *American Pharmacy's
Historical Collections* (second edition, 1965), has also noted that the
apothecary's "lore linked to the nostalgic, the curious and the beautiful,
appeals [as] strongly to the layman as to the pharmacist." Through
personal experience in museum work since September 1959, when I
joined the Smithsonian Institution as curator of the Division of Medical
Sciences, my awareness of this public appeal of health museums has
been sharpened and articulated. Some of the reasons for public interest
in pharmacy and health museums are obvious. Each family at one time
or another uses pharmaceutical compounds in seeking to preserve or
restore health and cure diseases. And as long as these needs are
present, then there will always be a demand for pharmaceutical prepara-

tions and professional and technical services. As long as the pharmacist plays an important and recognizable role in his community, his shop, tools, utensils, and the vessels in which he prepares, keeps, or dispenses his medications will be of interest. The pharmacist is a part of the health-care team, whether located in a hosptial, in a clinic, or in a rural or urban community pharmacy. This shop was, and in some respects still is, a meeting place for people. Many pharmacies in times past in North America made history when their proprietors entertained and developed friendships with leading contemporaries who left their impact on the history of the New World.

Over two decades have passed since I first became associated with the history of pharmacy, with special interest in the tools and equipment employed in the apothecary art and its manufacturing techniques and its heritage. Through acquaintance and dedication, I learned to love and appreciate these relics of the past with their aesthetic charm and intriguing qualities. Much can be learned from the study of artifacts. Our appreciation of past discoveries and contributions in science, technology, and the arts is enhanced as we see reflected in such artifacts the skill, craftmanship, and knowledge of pioneer scientists, inventors, and artists. Museums serve to link us with our ancestors and the products of their hands, minds, and wills.

It never fails to amaze me how these fragile artifacts bridge the gulf of centuries and show the interrelationship between cultures and peoples of many lands, their needs and aspirations, as well as the things they utilize in everyday living. They also expose connections between the belief and actions of people of varied backgrounds, so that we can see similarities in the action of a primitive mother who hangs a "protective" amulet around her child's neck and a contemporary mother in a highly civilized community who takes her child to a clinic for a prophylactic inoculation or vaccination. It further establishes our identity with the great worldwide human family. Indeed, the cultural history of North America is relatively recent if compared with that of ancient Egypt or Mesopotamia, where an excavated perfume vase or a scarab could have been the property of a person who outdated King Nebuchadnezzar of old Babylon, or who witnessed the construction of the Great Pyramids near Memphis in the land of the Nile.

It is rewarding for me to see such enthusiasm and appreciation for health museums in other countries mirroring their own achievements and medico-pharmaceutical practices and folklores. In this respect, several museums in Europe, Asia, Africa, Australia, and South America could be mentioned and from each we can learn much, especially when they collectively reflect the cultures of many peoples and lands with whom our own has reacted and continually interrelated. In recognizing other cultures, our appreciation of our own becomes the more lively and real. For further information on this theme, see my *Temples of the Muses and a History of Pharmacy Museums* (Tokyo: The Naito Foundation, 1972), pp. 4-88.

Every object or class of artifacts in a pharmacy museum has a story of its own. For example, the mortar and pestle can be traced back to the earliest civilizations; they have been used through the millenia not only in pharmacy and medicine, but also to prepare such things as food, cosmetics, and chemicals. In various times and cultures, they have been crafted of a wide range of materials from stone and alabaster to brass and iron to ceramics and glass and were often designed to reflect not only a specific period of history, but the status of the pharmacist within it. Other artifacts also have their fascinating traditions: the scales, weights and measures, the drug jars, the pill tile, the show globe, the distilling apparatus, and the crucible. We can also include paintings and prints of aesthetic value. But to discuss the history of these objects would carry us beyond the scope of this guidebook. Interested readers may find further help in the listing of published literature at the end of this guide.

As we enter the third century of the independence of the United States of America and the second of the dominion of Canada, we look expectantly to greater efforts at keeping the tradition and history of pharmacy alive and appreciated.

As the profession reaches in the future for higher goals, liberating itself from commercial and political entanglements, it should increase and sharpen its dedication to and understanding of the heritage of pharmacy. To create and increase such understanding is our primary, if humble, purpose for this guidebook which is dedicated to all those who appreciate and serve pharmacy.

S.K.H.

Pharmacy Museums and Exhibitions in the United States

The following entries are arranged alphabetically according to states and then to cities and towns within each state as well as the District of Columbia and Puerto Rico.

ALABAMA

Birmingham

Alabama Museum of Health Science
Lister Hill Library of the Health Sciences
1700 Eighth Avenue South
University of Alabama (in Birmingham)
University Station 35294
(205) 934-4475
Managed by the University of Alabama in Birmingham.

8:30 A.M. – 4:30 P.M.   Monday–Friday

Free

A large hall with exhibitions on pharmaceutical tools, drug bottles, medical and dental equipment, nursing and opthalmological artifacts, together with documents, photographs, memorabilia, and archival material related to the health professions and practice in the state of Alabama. In an adjacent hall is the Lawrence Reynolds Medico-Historical Library which includes rare books and archives.

Jacksonville

Dr. J.C. Francis Medical Museum
100 Gayle Street 36265
(205) 435-5247 / 7203
Located one block west of U.S. Highway 278 and Town Square.
Managed by the State of Alabama Historical Commission, 75
    Monroe Street, Montgomery, Alabama 36104. (204) 832-6621

11 A.M. – 3 P.M.	Saturday
1 P.M. – 4 P.M.	Sunday
Telephone for special appointment	

Free

The museum and grounds are owned by the state of Alabama, Alabama Historical Commission, and operated under the auspices of the General John H. Forney Historical Society, Inc. The museum was dedicated and opened to the public on March 21, 1974, when a marker in memory of Dr. Francis was unveiled by his great-grandson.

The restored rectangular structure, a quaint functional building, consists of two rooms—an apothecary shop in front leading into a doctor's office in the rear. The building was constructed about 1850 in the American national style architecture and has a pediment front porch supported by four Doric columns.

It was occupied by Dr. Francis for almost forty of his fifty-four years of practice as a family doctor in Jacksonville and is possibly the only building of its kind and function in northeast Alabama preserved from that era to this day.

On display in the museum are apothecary jars and medicine bottles, a plantation first-aid kit, surgical instruments, and various medication containers similar to those used or dispensed to clients more than a century ago. In addition, other period furnishings, scales, apothecary tools, journals, and books of the 1820 to the 1870s period are exhibited.

ARIZONA

Tucson

Arizona Pharmacy Museum
123 Pharmacy–Microbiology Building
College of Pharmacy, The University of Arizona 85721
(602) 626-1427 / 4429
Managed by the University of Arizona.

| By appointment | Monday–Friday |

Free

This well-planned university museum (founded 1966) comprises three exhibitions.

The W. Roy Wayland Memorial Foyer on pharmaceutical history with pharmaceutical manufacturing tools at the center. Wayland wrote Arizona's pharmacy law, and his original pharmacy started at Solomonville in 1903. The exhibit includes a materia-medica box with 288 hinged-lid windowed tin containers for identifying crude drugs, a physician's authentic desk and chair, plus two wall cases with tools of the apothecary, caricatures, and photographs.

The apothecary shop, a replica of an 1875 "botica" of territorial southwestern United States, contains authentic pictures, tools, and fixtures.

Period room of the 1920s, furnished with various tools of the apothecary, supplies, and fixtures. It displays jars and medicinal bottles, as well as books and archival material assembled and donated by pharmacist Jesse Hurlbut (licensed 1915) and his wife. On display also are illuminated show globes, a marble-top wrapping counter, posters, an iron settee for patrons, a mirrored soda fountain back bar as well as frontal fixture, slot- and hand-operated ice-cream machines, a Parke, Davis and Company materia-medica chest, tobacco cutter, cork press, scales, and herb, spices, and other crude drug containers as well as medico-pharmaceutical books and archives of historical interest.

ARKANSAS

Morrilton

Baker Drug Store Gift Shop
Route 3   72110
(501) 727-5427
Take Interstate 40, to Highway 9 S, then 154 W, Petit Jean
   Mountain, 14 miles from Morrilton. Owned and operated by the
   Museum of Automobiles; Buddy Holtzeman, director.

10 A.M. – 5 P.M.   daily, except Christmas

$2 admission to the automobile show and gift shop

Original fixtures were ordered by Dr. F.E. Baker to be custom built in Saint Louis, Missouri, in 1902 and shipped to Stamps, Arkansas. The store's decor and oak shelves are installed as they had been at their original location. Exhibited are medicinal bottles, a marble-top operational soda fountain with ornamental back bar, prescription inventory, glass display cases, and period ceiling fans. After Baker's death in 1949, his nephew Seth W. Baker and his wife operated the store until 1967 when it was dismantled at Stamps and moved to its new quarters. This exhibition, designed to provide a glimpse of the lively pages of pharmacy's "good old days," opened to the public in 1975 through a Rockefeller donation.

CALIFORNIA

Bakersfield

Carlock Apothecary Shop Exhibition
Kern County Museum's Pioneer Village
3801 Chester Avenue 93301
(805) 861-2132
Located about 100 miles north of Los Angeles in the southern end
of the San Joaquin Valley. Owned and administered by County of
Kern Board of Supervisors, state of California; Richard C.
Bailey, director.

8:00 A.M. – 3:30 P.M.	Monday–Friday
10:00 A.M. – 3:30 P.M.	Saturday, Sunday, and holidays

Adults, $1.00; children, 75¢

The original fixtures were built by Marion Carlock in 1890 and were
donated by his daughter. The exhibition opened to the public in 1957 in
this pioneering village with displays and artifacts dating from about 1880
to 1930. The apothecary furnishings include patent medicines (from
Ayer's Sarsaparilla to Pinkham's Pink Pills), herb containers, show
globes, drug jars, and prescription rack. Among over sixty other exhibitions and buildings is a doctor's office also opened in 1957 with furnishings including rolltop desk, operating table, machine for generating
static electricity, X-ray machine, a glass cabinet with surgical tools, an
early microscope, medicine kit, and pill case (arranged by Dr. R.E.
Scherb). There is also a dentist's office with dental chairs, foot drills,
X-ray machines, dentures, and dental instruments (donated in 1957 by
A. Kruger and the families of the late Drs. Glen Patton and H. Rade-
macher, dentists). These three exhibits beside others in Pioneer Village
provide a nostalgic view of central California in its pioneering days.

Buena Park

Knott's Berry Farm Drug Store
8039 Beach Boulevard 90620
Located two miles off the Santa Ana Freeway and about one mile
from Highway 91. Owned and operated by the Knott's Berry
Farm and Ghost Town & Western Trail Museum, founded 1956;
(714) 827-1776; Tracy Earlywine (information center).

Summer

10 A.M. – 6 P.M.	Monday–Friday
10 A.M. – midnight	Saturday
10 A.M. – 9 P.M.	Sunday

Winter

9 A.M. – 11 P.M.	Monday, Tuesday, Friday
9 A.M. – 1 P.M.	Saturday
9 A.M. – noon	Sunday

(Closed Wednesday and Thursday)

Adults, $1.00; children (to 11 years), 25¢

The original Ghost Town was developed and expanded since 1940 by Walter Knott (born 1889). Intended as an integral part of the Berry Farm experience and adventure and to pay homage to the pioneering spirit and love for the "old west." Initially an 1868 gold-trail hotel that contains a covered-wagon show, it was dismantled from near Prescott, Arizona, and moved here when many other authentic buildings were restored, including exhibits, log cabins, a modern colorful fiesta village, and a duplicate of Independence Hall. All exhibitions were reinstalled on a 150-acre farm. Of special interest is the "Pharmacy Display" representing an apothecary shop front in a general store. It exhibits a prescription department, stocks of medicinal bottles, tools, and artifacts of the apothecary art utilized in the "old west" from the 1860s to the end of the century and is typical of California's mining communities of this era. Another important exhibit is the dental office of Dr. Lamuel Walker with period equipment and tools.

Columbia

Columbia State Historic Park Drugstore
State Street, Columbia State Historic Park
P.O. Box 151   95310
(209) 532-4301
Managed by The Columbia State Historic Park; N. E. Power, area
    manager.

8:30 A.M. – 4:30 P.M.   daily; later in summer and on weekends

Free

The drugstore was presented to the state in 1957 by the California Pharmaceutical Association. It was licensed as a permanent display-only pharmacy museum of the gold-rush period by the Department of Professional and Vocational Standards. It depicts a California pharmacy of the late-nineteenth century with stock and fixtures, and an elegant mortar sign. Another park exhibit on Main Street depicts a Chinese (medicinal) Herb Shop of the period 1852–1870.

Los Angeles

The Upjohn Pharmacy Exhibition
California Museum of Science and Industry
Exhibition Park, 700 State Drive 90037
(213) 749-0101
Managed by the California Museum of Science and Industry
(founded 1880), and owned by the state of California; William J.
McCann, director.

10 A.M. – 5 P.M.   daily, except New Year's Day, Thanksgiving, and
Christmas

Free

This outstanding collection was first displayed for many years by the
Upjohn Company in Disneyland at Anaheim, California, before it was
donated to the museum. Supplemented by the museum's collection of
pharmaceutical equipment, it is one of the finest and most comprehensive pharmacy exhibitions in the western region. Included in the display
are show globes, mortars and pestles, scales and weights, medicinal
bottles, patent medicines, microscopes, tools, and drug containers.

San Diego

Witfeld Old Town Drug Store Museum
2482 San Diego Avenue 92110
(714) 298-2482
Owned and operated together with the Original Whaley House
(dating about 1857) by the Historical Shrine Foundation.

10 A.M. – 4 P.M.   Wednesday–Sunday

Free

In conjunction with the bicentennial of the establishment of the Mission
San Diego de Alcalan in June 1769 by Fra. Junípero Serra, the museum
was inaugurated in 1969 under the direction of Mrs. James Reading in
cooperation with the San Diego County and Southern California Pharmaceutical Associations. The museum is named after the pharmaceutical–chemist Gustavus Witfeld (also spelled Witfield and Wittfield) who
was born near what was then Cologne, Prussia, on January 27, 1825. He
became the city's first druggist in 1868 and died there on September 15,
1894. The original building was restored on the Whaley House grounds
and displays original furnishings; pharmaceutical implements; glass and
ceramic containers; pill, suppository, and tablet machines; soap cutter;
and percolators (from the 1850s to the 1880s).

A doctor's clinic with period equipment and tools is also attached to the Drug Store.

Adjacent to the museum is a botanical garden with spice herbs reminescent of a bygone era. (See E.W. Stieb, "The past recaptured, *"Pharmacy in History,* 18 (1976), p. 31, with acknowledged thanks to Edward S. Brady and Mrs. Marilyn Hall).

Stockton

The Holden Drug Company Exhibit
Victory Park, 1201 North Pershing 95203
(209) 462-4116 / 1566
Managed by The Pioneer Museum and Haggin Galleries; Raymond
   W. Hillman, curator of history.

1:30 – 5:00 P.M.   Tuesday–Sunday

Free

The 1870s exhibit of pharmaceutical equipment, stock, and fixtures are part of the E.S. Holden drugstore with additions dating from the late-nineteenth century. It is part of a gallery of store interiors within this art and history museum.

Stockton

The Lovotti Majolica Collection (Exhibition)
Wing A, Room 107, School of Pharmacy
University of the Pacific, 751 Brookside Road 95207
(209) 946-2561
Owned by the University of the Pacific at Stockton.

Open during school hours (eleven months of the year) by first
   contacting the Dean's Office

Free

The collection, a gift from pharmacist Carl D. Lovotti of San Francisco, consists of 55 majolica pieces of drug jars, plates, flasks, pitchers, and plaques from Castelli, Savona, Urbino, and Faenza dating from the fifteenth through the eighteenth centuries. The collection is displayed in mahogany showcases acquired from a nineteenth-century pharmacy in Fresno, California.

COLORADO

Central City

Best-Daugherty-Springer Historic Pharmacy
Bayless General Store
107 Eureka Street 80427
(303) 583-5313
Owned and operated by Roscoe and Carole Bayless.

9:00 A.M. – 5:30 P.M.   Monday–Saturday

Free

Apparently Colorado's oldest continuously operated drugstore, it is on what was considered the "richest square mile on earth." It was established in 1861 by pharmacist Hayes to supply drugs and mill chemicals to gold-rush miners in a city that became a cultural and trade center in the area. Three years later, it was purchased by John Best, a graduate of the New York College of Pharmacy, who continued to dispense medications and chemicals. He also provided health-care services for residents and visitors of Gilpin County before and after the fire of 1874 which destroyed a great part of the "oldest and most historic mining camp in America," including the pharmacy shop. After rebuilding it with new enlarged fixtures and stock, Best was succeeded in 1887 by druggist Llewellyn P. Davies who enlarged the business greatly and started pharmaceutical manufacturing. One of his many specialties, which enjoyed great popularity—samples of which are now on exhibit—was "The Miner Drink." He advertised it in the local newspaper as being "especially compounded after months of careful study, for the benefits of the miners, for relieving the bronchial tubes, and preserving the lungs after inhaling powder, smoke, dust, bad air, etc., besides being a strong and invigorating tonic."

In 1933 the drugstore was purchased and operated by pharmacist Frank Daugherty and his wife who was actually the first to give special attention to collecting historical artifacts and to preserving the original structure. Daugherty was succeeded in 1947 by pharmacist George N. Springer and his wife, Kathleen, who promoted and maintained a museum-like interior for public view until their retirement in early 1976 when the store passed to the hands of the present owners.

On display are elegant fixtures and a winding staircase with Victorian woodwork dating from 1874, prescription records of the mid-1880s, patent drugs and trademarked medicine bottles on original mahogony shelves, hand-blown glassware, show globes of the mid-nineteenth century, scales, mortars, crucibles, botanical drugs, cigar and majestic show cases, kerosene lamps, pill and suppository machines, and other apothecary tools as well as pre- and post-1900 pharmaceutical specialties. See K. Springer et al., "An Historic Pharmacy," *Pharmacy in History,* 16 (1974), pp. 97-101; and H.B. Rames, "The Pharmacy," *Modern Pharmacy,* 35 (September 1950), pp. 25-29.

Fair Play

Fair Play Park Pharmacy
South Park City Museum
P.O. Box 460   80440
(303) 836-2387
Affiliated with South Park Historical Foundation, Inc.; Carol A.
Davis, general manager, and Eric Swanson, curator.

9 A.M. – 5 P.M.	May 15–Memorial Day
9 A.M. – 7 P.M.	Memorial Day–Labor Day
9 A.M. – 5 P.M.	Labor Day–October 15

Adults, $2.00; children and senior citizens, 50¢; group rates are available.

This is a historic village museum founded in 1957 on the site of a post-Civil War mining town of about 1879 with collections dating from 1860 to 1920. It includes temporary exhibitions as well as twenty-five permanent exhibit buildings, including a pharmacy shop. It has an extensive collection of patent medicines.

Fort Garland

Old Fort Garland Restoration
P.O. Box 208   81133
(303) 379-3512
Owned by the State Historical Society of Colorado and operated
under the auspices of the Colorado Heritage Center, 1300
Broadway, Denver 80203; (303) 892-2136. Regional curator Bill
Hoagland and R.M. Doherty, curator-in-charge.

10 A.M. – 4 P.M.   daily, May 15–October 1

Adults, $1.50; children and senior citizens, 75¢; school groups, 25¢ each

This is a restoration of an historic fort once commanded by Kit Carson. The fort was active 1858–1883. The exhibit includes one case containing a Civil War medical field kit as well as medicinal containers, surgical and medical tools, and equipment representing the health profession in Colorado Territory during the Civil War period.

CONNECTICUT

Mystic

The H.R. Bringhurst Drug Store
Mystic Seaport 06355
(203) 536-2631
Located about ten miles east of New London on thirty-seven acres
of seashore grounds on the east bank of Mystic River (Mystic
Seaport is a reproduction of a late-nineteenth-century New
England coastal town). It is owned by Mystic Seaport Museum,
Inc.; public affairs representative, William North.

9 A.M. – 5 P.M.   daily, except Thanksgiving and Christmas. (Ships
and buildings on Seaport Street and Village Street are staffed
from May through October by attendants who serve as
interpreters.)

Adults, $7.00; children, $3.50 during summer months; $6.00 and
$3.00, respectively, in winter (tickets provide access to all
exhibition grounds, including buildings, ships, and lofts).

Set up in 1964, the drugstore and doctor's office were rearranged in
1975 to represent more accurately the 1870-1885 period. The restoration
centers around the century-old original fixtures of the store and medical
clinic of Dr. Joseph Bringhurst (1767-1834) and his son (1807-1880).
The father moved from Philadelphia, Pennsylvania, to Wilmington,
Delaware, in 1793 where he established a drugstore in connection with
his medical practice as was the custom in those days when the two
professions were sometimes practiced by the same person. The business
flourished further under the son, a practitioner. The fixtures were fitted
out with period pharmaceutical equipment and artifacts (1870s to 1900).

Displayed are fine examples of show globes, medicine bottles and
jars, mortars and pestles, weights and scales, leech jars, bleeder knife,
ear trumpet, glycerin dispenser, spices, dye cabinet and paint pigments,
pill tiles, powder folders, tincture presses, proprietries, kerosene-oil
dispenser, medicine kits and counters, posters, books, and archival
materials, as well as material to refurbish ships' medicine chests.

The restored structure was financed by the Davella Mills Foundation
and the Gorg Bell Manufacturing Company while the original fixtures
and utensils were donated by Smith, Kline and French Laboratories of
Philadelphia in 1953. Later, other items and donations were added
together with the adjacent doctor's period office with an old desk and
medical and dental tools.

New Canaan

The Monroe–Cody Drug Store
13 Oenoke Ridge 06840
(203) 966-1776
Owned by the New Canaan Historical Society.

9:30 A.M. – 12:30 P.M. and 2:00 P.M. – 4:30 P.M.
Tuesday – Saturday

Free

When Main Street was widened during the late summer of 1965, this town landmark was donated by the son and daughters of pharmacist James J. Cody to the Historical Society. The original patent-medicine store was established in 1845 by Samuel Cook Silliman. Doctors came here to dispense drugs. In 1854, it was sold to Lucius M. Monroe who installed the present fixtures, renovated the shop to improve its operation, and dispensed medicine himself to his customers. It was known then as the New Canaan Drug Store. In 1918, pharmacist Cody, who had been long associated with Monroe, bought it and directed the business until his death when his two daughters took charge until they donated its contents to the Historical Society. Here at the annex of the Town House, the elegant interior fixtures, apothecary tools, patent medicines, and advertisement signs are conveniently displayed, portraying a representative image of the pre-Civil War American drugstore.

New Haven

Streeter-Lewis Pharmacy Exhibition
333 Cedar Street 06510
(203) 436-2566
Owned and operated by the Yale Medical Library, Yale University.

8:30 A.M. – 5:00 P.M.   Monday – Friday

Free

The contents and furnishings from the Old and New Worlds in the pharmacy room are the gift of Dr. Edward Clark Streeter (1874–1947). The alcove has mostly American items (1845–1880, eastern Connecticut), including a tall herb cabinet dated 1880. Hand-blown American glasswares and pill machines are from Mystic and Hope Valley. The European faience and glasswares, mortars and drug jars (dating 1500–1800) are shelved in the main, largely Sicilian room. Also of pharmaceutical interest is the remarkable Streeter Collection of weights, balances, gold coin scales, and linear and bulk measures from the ancient civilizations to those of nineteenth-century Europe and America. These are displayed in special show cabinets donated by Wilmarth S. Lewis and his wife.

The exhibition is housed in the historical section of Yale Medical Library. The library also houses medical and surgical instruments, kits, saddle bags, slides, medals, bookplates, prints, drawings, and portraits. The collections of old books, manuscripts, incunabula, archival materials, and historical periodicals owe their origins in 1935 to Harvey Cushing and later his two friends—Arnold C. Kleb and John F. Fulton. Other artifacts include obstetrical forceps, scarificators, eyeglasses, microscopes, endoscopes, catheters, probes, vaporizers, atomizers, and kymographs.

Storrs

The Mogull Apothecary Collection
School of Pharmacy, The University of Connecticut 06268
(203) 429-3311
Owned and operated by the University of Connecticut School of
Pharmacy, office of the dean, Arthur E. Schwarting.

8:30 A.M. – 4:30 P.M.   Monday – Friday during school year and
summer, except holidays

Free

Donated in 1967 by Edith Smith Mogull in memory of her late husband, pharmacist Edward Mogull (d. 1963), whose interest in pharmacy's relics goes back to the 1940s. The collection includes drug jars, wooden and metal mortars and pestles, glass bottles, show globes, medico- pharmaceutical books including a copy of the first *United States Pharmacopoeia* of 1820 and other related pharmaceutical antiques, tools, and equipment. The collection is displayed in the hallways of the Pharmacy Research Institute building at the university.

Waterbury

The Mattatuck Apothecary Shop
199 West Main Street 06702
(203) 754-5500
Owned and operated by the Mattatuck Museum.

| 12 noon – 5 P.M. | Tuesday – Saturday |
| 2 P.M. – 5 P.M. | Sunday |

Free

This late-nineteenth century apothecary shop, within the Mattatuck Museum of Art, History, and Industry, holds original fixtures, period equipment, tools, and shelf wares brought from a pharmacy in Stoney Creek, Connecticut, with additions added later.

DISTRICT OF COLUMBIA

Washington

Armed Forces Medical Museum
6825 Sixteenth Street, N.W. 20306
(202) 576-2341
Located on the grounds of Walter Reed Army Medical Center.
Owned and managed by the Armed Forces Institute of Pathology, Department of Defense; officially established July 6, 1949, as a central diagnostic research and teaching center in pathological studies with the Health, Education and Welfare Department's Public Health Service.

12 noon – 6 P.M.   daily

Free

Founded by the United States Surgeon General of the Army, William A. Hammond, in 1862 in direct response to a desperate human need and was the first of its kind in North America.

From 1887 to 1969, it shared a magnificent red-brick building on the Mall next to the Smithsonian at Seventh Street and Independence Avenue, S.W., with the Army Medical Library (later the Armed Forces Medical Library and presently the National Library of Medicine), as conceived in the visionary plans of Dr. John Shaw Billings (director, 1865–1895). When the building was demolished, the museum collections were moved to their present quarters. The elaborate comprehensive exhibits were reopened to the public on May 2, 1971.

The exhibition displays pathological specimens, military and medical artifacts, and instruments which have been collected since the Civil War period. The museum is divided into four halls and archives and an auditorium.

History of Pharmacy and Health Halls
Division of Medical Sciences, Department of the History of Science
and Technology, National Museum of American History
(formerly National Museum of History and Technology),
Smithsonian Institution
12th and Constitution, N.W. 20560
(202) 357-2145

10:00 A.M. – 5:30 P.M.   daily, after Labor Day to April 1
10 A.M. – 9 P.M.   daily, April 1 through Labor Day

Free

Three types of exhibits are represented in the Hall of Pharmaceutical
History: (1) a platform showing the development of tools, machines,
and equipment used in the manufacture of dosage forms from
pharmaceutical preparations in the nineteenth century to the first

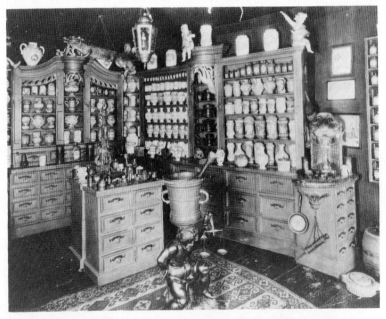

An apothecary museum which was reconstructed and displayed at the E.R.
Squibb and Sons headquarters in New York City between 1935–1944 with tools,
furnishings, and shelf ware. It is now on permanent loan to the Smithsonian
Institution's National Museum of American History (formerly the National Museum of History and Technology) in Washington, D.C.

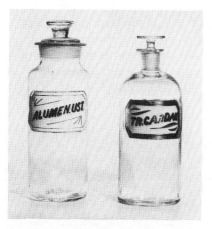

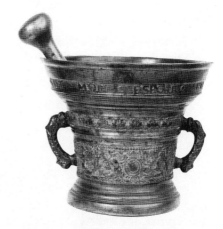

American glass drug bottles which are typical of the nineteenth century. The bottle on the left is called a "saltmouth;" the one on the right, a "tincture." Both have curved labels, typical of American bottles after 1860.

A 1615 Burgundian bronze mortar, inscribed "In God is my hope" in mixed Dutch and French jargon, is a classic example of high Renaissance decoration. It is part of the E.R. Squibb and Sons collection on display in the Smithsonian Institution.

quarter of the twentieth century; (2) special exhibit cases illustrating the evolution of the drug jar, mortars and pestles, equipment and specimens connected with the early development and manufacture of antibiotics and other drugs, and faith healing devices; (3) two pharmacy shop reconstructions.

Most of the baroque fixtures of the one shop had been a part of the eighteenth-century "Muenster Apotheke" of Freiburg im Breisgau in Germany. The shelf ware of glass, ceramic, porcelain and wood vessels and containers, as well as the tools and utensils range from the fifteenth through the nineteenth centuries. This unique and rather comprehensive collection is supplemented by rare pharmaceutical texts, edicts, prints, and franchises. The laboratory, or study room, shows authentic period furnishings, stuffed animals, and stained window glass. Acquired by E.R. Squibb and Sons (1932), the collection is on permanent exhibition through the courtesy of the American Pharmaceutical Association.

The second shop is an 1890 American drugstore. The original Victorian fixtures and the two prescription counters were donated in 1958 by pharmacist Michel H. Wagman of the Roach Drug Company, 8th and G Streets, S.E., Washington, D.C., established earlier by the O'Donnell family. The shelf ware, show globes and jars, patent medicines and posters, scales, ceramic and glass vessels and crude drug containers, tools, clock, prescription sign, and the lighted mortar and pestle sign are period pieces.

In addition, there are individual exhibits on medical and dental instruments and equipment, a corner of a hospital ward, X-ray tubes and machines, spectacles, faith and physical healing implements, and a bacteriology laboratory.

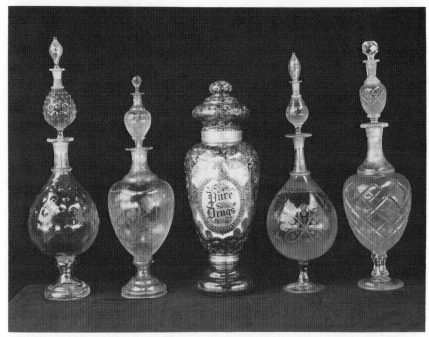

Late nineteenth-century American show globes and a display vase are in the Smithsonian Institution's collection. The vase in the center is inscribed "Pure Drugs" for advertising purposes. The two show globes on the extreme left and right are of Grecian type; the second and fourth are the pineapple type used for window exhibition using colored liquids and reflecting light.

Facing, top. The prescription section of an 1890 American drugstore displayed in the Smithsonian Institution's National Museum of American History (formerly the National Museum of History and Technology). Seen on the shelves are period chemicals, syrups, and drugs, as well as tools and light fixtures.

Facing, bottom. A restoration of an 1890 American drugstore is displayed with period furnishings and shelf ware from the Smithsonian's collection in the National Museum of American History (formerly the National Museum of History and Technology). The fixtures are authentic, with minor repairs, and come from a pharmacy shop which operated in the District of Columbia until the middle of this century.

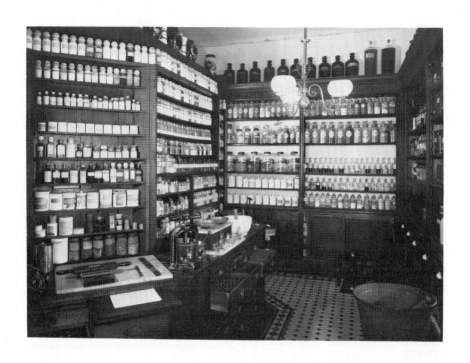

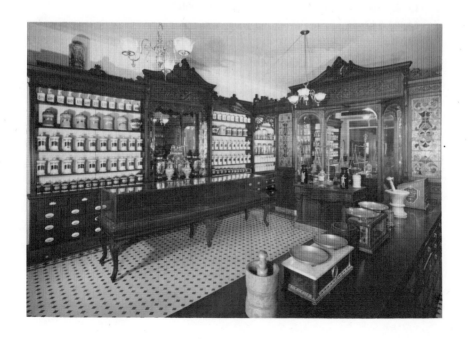

FLORIDA

Pensacola

Pensacola Historical Museum
405 South Adams Street (on Seville Square) 32501
(904) 433-1559
Owned and operated by Pensacola Historical Society; Ms. Sandra
Johnson, assistant curator.

9:00 A.M. – 4:30 P.M.   Monday – Saturday
Closed Sunday

Free

A display case devoted to pharmaceutical equipment and artifacts,
dental tools, medicine chests, and prescription books representing local
professional technology from the pre-Civil War period to 1940.

GEORGIA

Athens

Historical Pharmacy Exhibits
School of Pharmacy, University of Georgia
D.W. Brooks Drive at Green Street 30602
(404) 542-1911
Owned and managed by the University of Georgia.

8:30 A.M. – 4:30 P.M.   Monday – Friday
Appointments should be made with Prof. Douglas Johnson,
Pharmacology Department, or the Dean's Office.

Free

Eight panels display pharmaceutical themes and artifacts of historical
and professional interest. The exhibits rotate periodically.

Atlanta

Southern Pharmacy Exhibition
Mercer University
Southern School of Pharmacy
345 Boulevard North East 30312
(404) 688-6291
Owned and operated by the Mercer University; contact Dr.
Norman Franke or the Dean's Office.

9:00 A.M. – 4:30 P.M.   Monday – Friday, during school year

Free

A student lounge room has fixtures from an Atlanta drugstore of the early 1900s. Displayed on shelves are apothecary jars, proprietary or patent medicines, and the tools of the apothecary, including an iron mortar and pestle of the Revolutionary period.

Columbus

The Pemberton House and Apothecary
Historic House Museum
11 Seventh Street 31901
(404) 322-0756
Owned and operated by the Historic Columbus Foundation, Inc.,
    P.O. Box 5312   31906; Mrs. J.J.W. Biggers, Jr., executive
    director.

10 A.M. – 4 P.M.   Monday – Friday
Also part of Heritage Tour, 10 A.M., on Wednesdays and Saturdays
    from the Georgia Welcome Center on Victory Drive. A small fee
    is charged.

Free; donations accepted

This house was moved to this location from its original site at 1017 Third Avenue, and was restored to the simple four-room Victorian cottage it was in 1855 when it was occupied by Dr. John Styth Pemberton (1833–1888), a Georgia pharmacist–chemist. The out-building, originally the kitchen, has been furnished to resemble a "chemical laboratory" of that period in which Dr. Pemberton might have practiced his trade. Dr. Pemberton paid $1,950 for this house, his first purchased residence.

It was in Columbus in a chemical laboratory that Dr. Pemberton began preparing and dispensing his "cool, cordial and refreshing drinks" to his customers and regularly advertised them in the *Columbus Enquirer-Sun*. These "concoctions" and "draughts" often included one called "French Wine of Cocoa—ideal nerve tonic and stimulant," which was the forerunner of the internationally famous Coca-Cola Syrup and soft drink.

Dr. Pemberton and his family moved from Columbus to Atlanta where in 1887 he sold the secret of the Coca-Cola formula for $1,750 to pharmacist Asa G. Candler, founder of the Coca-Cola Company. Dr. Pemberton died in Atlanta in 1888. He is buried in historic Linwood Cemetery in Columbus, Georgia.

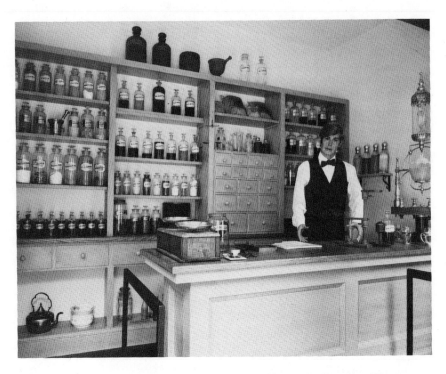

Display at the Pemberton Apothecary Shop in Columbus, Georgia. (Photo courtesy of the Historic Columbus Foundation, Inc.)

On display are period fixtures. Also displayed is a Charles Tuft soda fountain, one of two known in this country—the other is at the Smithsonian Institution—which featured several flavored syrups and mineral waters.

Other tools in the exhibit include a pill tile; a pill roller; spatulas for mixing ointments and salves; mortars and pestles; and medicinal, perfume, and Coca-Cola bottles. Recently acquired is the extensive Dr. Jesse L. Miller antique Coca-Cola Memorabilia Collection. See Charles Howard Candler, *Asa Griggo Candler* (Atlanta: Emory University Press, 1950), pages 134–159.

Lumpkin

Dr. Paullin's Office Exhibition
Westville Historic Handicrafts, Inc.
P.O. Box 1850   31815
(912) 838-6310

Owned and operated by the Westville Historic Handicrafts, Inc., in charge of Homer Moore.

10 A.M. – 5 P.M.	Monday – Saturday
1 P.M. – 5 P.M.	Sunday

Adults, $2.50; children, $1.00; senior citizens, $1.50. This fee entitles visitors to tour all thirty-three buildings, shops, and exhibitions at Westville Village restoration.

This is a restoration of the office and apothecary shop of Dr. William L. Paullin established in 1845 in Fort Gaines, Georgia, moved and reconstructed at the Westville Village grounds for public view. It contains original period furnishings including medical equipment, medicine kits and tools, dental instruments, herbal charts, desks, and a collection of mortars and pestles.

Lumpkin

The Hatchett Drug Store Museum
Stewart County 31815
(912) 323- 2612
Owned and operated by the Westville Historic Commission.

1 P.M. – 5 P.M.	daily, June – September
1 P.M. – 5 P.M.	weekends, October – May

$1

This is a drugstore restoration of an original established and operated in Fort Gaines, Georgia, from 1880 – 1957. The fixtures and equipment including shelves refurbished with medicinal bottles, tools of the apothecary, prescriptions, Dr. James Marion Hatchett's (1924–1894) M.D. diploma, date of graduation, and other memorabilia as well as pictures and books which were moved to Westville. The entire exhibition is designed as a functioning living-history village of authentically restored buildings depicting handicrafts and culture of Georgia's most romantic era in the mid-nineteenth century.

Savannah

Solomon's Pharmacy Exhibit
337 Bull Street 31401
(912) 232- 8169
Owned and operated by pharmacist Roy G. Thomas, proprietor.

8:30 A.M. – 5:30 P.M.	Monday – Friday
8:30 A.M. – 1:00 P.M.	Saturday

Free

This is a restoration of pharmacist Abraham A. Solomon's pharmacy which he established at Savannah in 1845, and moved to Bull Street in 1913 together with some period memorabilia including a letter from Gen. Robert E. Lee about a personal prescription. At this time, the present elegant mahogony fixtures and fourteen leaded stained-glass globes and showcases were installed. This still-functioning drugstore was purchased in 1974 by the present owner who intends to keep it with its historic section as a part of his growing pharmacy practice in this historic district of the city near the Scottish Rite Temple. Other pharmaceutical objects include patent medicines, tin, wood, glass, and ceramic drug containers, cash register, mortars and pestles, and the Solomon's Bitters associated with this enterprise since the mid-nineteenth century.

ILLINOIS

Chicago

Early American Apothecary Shop
Main Floor, International Museum of Surgical Science and Hall of
    Fame
1524 North Lake Shore Drive 60610
(312) 642-3555
Owned and operated by the International College of Surgeons, 1516
    North Lake Shore Drive, George F. Smith, M.D., director.

10 A.M. – 4 P.M.   Tuesday – Sunday (closed Monday)

Free

Among thirty-two rooms and halls displaying artifacts, models, instruments, illustrations of the history of surgery and therapy, and the story of mankind's continuing struggle against suffering and disease, is a reconstructed late nineteenth-century drugstore. Many of its fixtures and pieces of equipment are authentic, dating back to the last quarter of the nineteenth century. These were furnishings and artifacts preserved from an 1873 drugstore owned by Charles W. Sackett (d. 1917) and Fred C. Taber (d. 1880) of Addison, New York. Additional fixtures, equipment, and merchandise came from the apothecary shop of Dr. Uriah C. Jones (about 1882) of Breda, Iowa, and donations were made by Mr. and Mrs. Maurice E. Miller of Ithaca, New York, and Lee Alport of Elmwood Park, Illinois.

In this spacious exhibition are two prescription counters, display cases, period lighting fixtures and shelf ware, a do-it-yourself medical

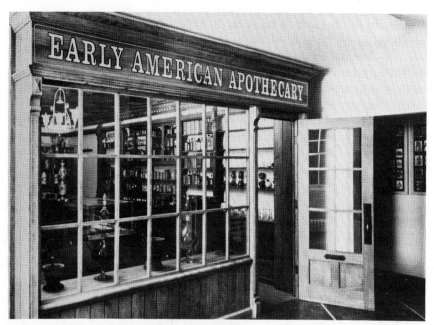

The Early American Apothecary Shop (1873) at the International Museum of Surgical Science and Hall of Fame, International College of Surgeons at Chicago, Illinois.

kit, jars and tools of the apothecary, and drawers labeled with the names of stored herbs. Also on display are show globes, scales and weights, patent medicines and "quack remedies" advertisements, sanitary and sundry items, pharmacy records, registration certificates, and a manikin of a practicing pharmacist. The exhibit was inaugurated on November 30, 1966, under the auspices of Charles R. Walgreen, Jr.

Chicago

Museum and History Laboratory
College of Pharmacy Building
833 South Wood Street 60680
(312) 996-7190
Owned and operated by the University of Illinois College of
Pharmacy; Marvin Weinstein, curator.

Monday – Friday, during school year and by appointment

Free

Objects on shelves and in late-nineteenth-century cabinets are arranged according to the purpose of the pharmaceutical preparations and the utility of the specimens exhibited. These were donated by Illinois pharmacists or their heirs and consist of tools of the apothecary, cosmetics, medicated soaps and tampons, plasters, patent medicines, tin herb cans, scales, mortars, and books and pharmaceutical catalogs, archives, and registers. Some of the registers and prescriptions go back to the 1840s, before the founding of the Chicago College of Pharmacy in 1859.

Chicago

The Old Apothecary Shop
Medical Balcony, Museum of Science and Industry
57th Street and South Lake Shore Drive 60637
(312) 684-1414
Located along Lake Michigan on fourteen acres in Jackson Park on Chicago's southside.
Owned and operated by the Museum of Science and Industry.

9:30 A.M. – 5:30 P.M.	daily, May – Labor Day
9:30 A.M. – 4:00 P.M.	Monday – Friday, balance of year
9:30 A.M. – 5:30 P.M.	Saturday, Sunday, and holidays, except Christmas

Free

Occupying the reconstructed Fine Arts Building of the 1893 Columbia Exposition, the classically architectured museum opened in 1933. Oriented toward advances in pure and applied sciences and industrial technology, it displays several exhibits on health and biology; a giant 16-foot walk-through human heart, hatching of live baby chicks, and a full-size transparent manikin of a woman to show bodily function.

Most relevant, however, is the old apothecary-shop exhibition, a nostalgic replica of a mid-nineteenth-century American drugstore. It was named after Philo Carpenter (1805-1885), a pioneer Chicago pharmacist, philanthropist, and social reformer. It includes fixtures and pharmacy tools of the second half of the nineteenth century with shelf ware, genuine horehound drops, cod-liver oil, patent medicines, drug jars, cosmetics, soap, sponges, chamois skins, hearing aids, chest protectors, trusses, spectacles, an assortment of sachet and complexion powders, and prescription books of the 1870s. Most of the collection on display was assembled and donated by Dr. Christianson of Chicago in the 1930s.

Hinsdale

Health Education Center Exhibition
The Robert Crown Center for Health Education
21 Salt Creek Lane 60521
(312) 325-1900.
Owned and operated by the above center; Arthur C. Wiscombe,
executive director.

9 A.M. – 3 P.M.	Monday – Friday, mid-September–mid-June for school groups only
3 P.M. – 4:30 P.M.	Monday – Friday, other than school groups
9 A.M. – 2 P.M.	Monday – Friday, mid-June–mid-September Closed on national holidays

$1.25; class groups by reservation only and at established
instructional program rates.

It was founded and managed by the inventor-engineer, Charles
Kettering, and designated as a family foundation from 1958 to 1969.
Since then, it became a nonprofit organization supported by membership, admission fees, and voluntary contributions to the Center represented by the Health Education Institute. The exhibition represents a
dynamic, bold venture in the field of health education, family planning,
drug information for the prevention of abuse and the improvement of
diet and medication therapy, environmental quality, and better health
and family living habits. Among the attractions is "Valeda," the
transparent talking lady which demonstrates human body organs and
their functions through an audio-visual arrangement geared toward
group viewing and guided tours; the brain; and nervous system. The
animated exhibits on blood circulation, how life begins or human
reproduction, attempt to explain the anatomy and physiology of the
human body, its growth and development. There are assorted collections
of medications, drug containers, and tools; lectures and films related to
drug abuse are given periodically.

Peoria

Bogard Pharmacy Restoration
Bogard Drugs no. 2
3506 North Prospect Road 61603
(309) 685-7636
Owned and managed by Richard H. Bogard, pharmacist–proprietor, and chairman of the board of Bogard Drug Stores.

9 A.M. – 8 P.M.	Monday – Friday
9 A.M. – 6 P.M.	Saturday
9 A.M. – 4 P.M.	Sunday

Free

Richard and Mary Bogard have collected pharmaceutical antiques for the last quarter of a century. The oak fixtures and some of the artifacts were acquired from a drugstore in Centerville, Iowa, in 1974, and date from about 1900. The display is designed to depict and preserve pharmaceutical heritage in objects, especially the early part of this century, and includes period tools of the apothecary, show globes, tin and glass wares, showcases and kits, trading cards, patent medicines and books.

INDIANA

Evansville

The Hugh McGary Memorial Exhibit
The Evansville Museum of Arts and Sciences
411 S.E. Riverside Drive 47713
(812) 425-2406
Located on the banks of the Ohio River.
Owned and operated by the Evansville Museum of Arts and Sciences; Mr. John W. Streetman III, director, and F.P. Martin, research curator.

10 A.M. – 5 P.M.	Tuesday – Saturday
Noon – 5 P.M.	Sunday (closed Monday)

Free

A reproduction of the office and apothecary shop of Dr. William Morton Elliott, who was graduated from Evansville Medical College in 1853, with figures of the doctor and a ten-year-old girl. It evokes memories of medico-pharmaceutical practice in the city during the second half of the nineteenth century. The exhibit was named in honor of Hugh McGary, who in 1812 purchased 200 acres which later became the site of the incorporated town of Evansville.

In the exhibit are displayed drug jars, medicine bottles, show globes, microscopes, nursing bottles, and tools of the apothecary, including pill tiles and machines, konseals, cork press, measures, mortars and pestles, scales, drug mills, and suppository molds. It also contains medical and surgical equipment, including scarificators, syringes, lancets, amputation kit, splints, and obstetric tools, as well as Dr. Elliott's medical diploma, textbooks, class cards, his thesis, and a letter of recommendation signed by members of the faculty of the Evansville Medical College. The exhibit was developed and sponsored by the Vanderburgh County Medical Society, the Evansville Museum of Arts and Sciences, and by a group from Mead Johnson and Company of Evansville.

Evansville

Mead Johnson's Antique Pediatric Exhibition
2404 West Pennsylvania Street 47721
(812) 426-6428
Owned and operated by Mead Johnson and Company;
R.M. Eckels, director of public affairs.

7:30 A.M. – 4:00 P.M.   Monday – Friday

Free

A fine collection of pediatric antiques in one large exhibit case installed in the lobby of the administration building. The company was started in Jersey City, New Jersey, in 1905 by Edward Mead Johnson. The company moved to Evansville in 1915 and merged with Bristol–Myers Company in 1967. It was a chemical manufacturing plant, then turned to medical and sterile surgical supplies, and eventually became a leader in the field of infant nutrition. Mead Johnson developed an interest in collecting pediatric and pharmaceutical objects related to child health and nutritional products, which are represented in the display.

Indianapolis

Hook's Historical Drug Store and Pharmacy Museum
Indiana State Fairgrounds
1202 East 38th Street 46205
(317) 924-1503
Operated by Hook Drugs, Inc.

11 A.M. – 5 P.M.   daily

Free

A vast collection of American pharmacy artifacts, drugstore and soda fountain memorabilia is housed in this nineteenth-century drugstore and museum, featuring rare ornate carved furnishings built in 1849.

Opened in 1966, the large, authentic exhibit features fine early pharmacy wares from England, France, and Germany. An 1880 Lippincott soda-water apparatus provides a unique setting for a working soda fountain that boasts the finest chocolate soda in Indiana. Many old-time candies, tobaccos, toiletries, and novelties are for sale.

Lilly Center Exhibition and Archives
893 South Delaware Street 46206
(317) 261-2771
Owned and operated by Eli Lilly and Company, 307 East McCarty
Street (46206); Mrs. Anita Martin, archivist, and A.F. Martell,
guest-relations manager.

9 A.M. – 4 P.M.   Monday, Tuesday, Thursday, and Friday
11 A.M. – 4 P.M.   Wednesday
Evenings by appointment

Free

Lilly Center graphically portrays, in seven major exhibits, within a large
exhibit hall, the company's diversified interests in pharmaceuticals, agri-
chemicals, packaging, cosmetics, and animal health products. Extensive
exhibits on diabetes and antibiotics are also included, in addition to the
company's capsule manufacturing operation.

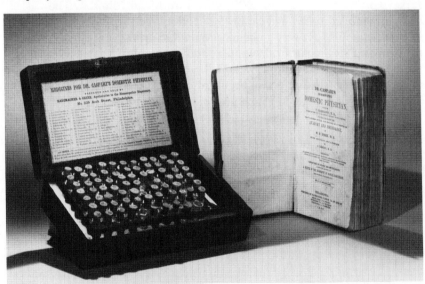

This homeopathic medicine case is typical of many on the market around the
turn of the century. It is shown with an 1852 copy of Dr. Caspari's homeopathic
Domestic Physician which was used for home treatment. (Courtesy of the Eli
Lilly and Company's archives)

A special "Lilly" room is devoted to mementos and history of the Lilly family associated with the firm and is adjacent to several corporate archival displays. The major theme is an illustration of the story of the company, its products, and its widespread diversified operations. The visitor can learn of the discovery, development, production, and application of the company's pharmaceutical and other preparations and specialties listed above.

Mitchell

Spring Mill Village Apothecary Shop
Spring Mill State Park, RR. 2, State 60   47446
(812) 849-4129
Owned and operated by the Department of Natural Resources, the
   state of Indiana; Mrs. Ruth Williams, village supervisor

9 A.M. – 5 P.M.   daily, April – November

Free

A restored pioneer village consisting of a dozen buildings including a general store, a museum, and a frontier apothecary shop with fixtures, equipment, and tools of the pre-Civil War period (some of the glasswares and utensils are of a later vintage).

Nashville

The 1900 John A. Hook Drug Store
State Road 46 East 47448
(812) 988-7463
Operated by Hook Drugs, Inc.

9 A.M. – 9 P.M.   daily
9 A.M. – 7 P.M.   Sunday

Free

Actual furnishings from the first Hook's Drug Store have been reassembled in this quaint Brown County setting as an operating turn-of-the-century drugstore. The traditional pharmacy and drugstore memorabilia are displayed in a living setting, where many old-time candies, toiletries, and tobaccos are for sale. A vintage marble soda fountain offers a variety of confections, including ice cream sodas made the old-fashioned way.

IOWA

Algona

Drug Store Exhibition
P.O. Box 370   50511
Highway 18 West
(515) 295-2461
Owned and operated by the Druggists Mutual Insurance Company.

8:00 A.M. – 4:30 P.M.   Monday – Friday and by special
appointment

Free

The idea of establishing the exhibition was initiated by the company (as plans were made for a new office building in early 1970) with the hope that tribute could be paid by re-creating a part of our heritage. The company was founded in 1909 by A. Falkenhainer who served for a number of years as secretary of the Iowa Board of Pharmacy in the aftermath of the destruction by fire of his drugstore in Titonka in 1902.

The reconstructed exhibition, opened to the public in 1972, was patterned after period-type stores at the turn-of-the-century when the insurance company was founded.

Off the main lobby, a 26 x 26-foot room with an oak floor was assigned for the exhibition. It is designed for the purpose of preserving the historic role of pharmacy in Iowa and other midwestern states with artifacts and fixtures donated by policy holders. They include a reception desk with the original marble top and an 1880 wrapping counter; a 1909 jump-spark cigar lighter; Scup matchbook dispenser (matchbooks sold then for one cent); a materia-medica teaching kit, containing 161 small boxes of crude drugs and herbs ordered from Eli Lilly & Company; eyeglasses and an 1890 optometrist's kit; rye-ole (soda) fountain vase-holder for cola, complete with a back bar, table, and wire-back chairs; and a "Diamond Dye" case. Among other objects and sundries are glass-labeled shelf bottles, proprietary remedies, scales, perfumes, baby supplies, and many other items as well as various tools of the apothecary arranged in an elegant setting. Uniquely, this exhibit is installed to dramatize the fact that this insurance company was organized and established by pharmacists and is still maintained exclusively by and for pharmacists and similar health professionals.

Furthermore, other displays and pictures throughout the new building tell the story of pharmacy as it was in Titonka and the Midwest about 1900.

Charles City

Legel's Drug Store Restoration
107 North Main Street 50616
(515) 228-3563 / 4234
Located three blocks off the Hiawatha Pioneer trail, Highways 18,
   218, and 14 at the Court House corner. Owned and operated by
   the Floyd County Historical Society; Mark E. Ferguson,
   president.

1:30 P.M. – 4:30 P.M.	Thursday – Sunday, from first Sunday of May–last Sunday of September; other times by appointment

Adults, 50¢; children, 10¢; yearly membership, $1.00

It is a part of the Floyd County Historical Society Museum dedicated to preserving the county's heritage, including a drug and grocery business establishment that started in 1873. The business was bought in 1884 by John G. Legel and it remained in the family until 1961 when the building, the original furnishings, and the entire collections of pharmaceutical antiques were donated to the society's museum which opened in 1962. Besides the soda fountain and the prescription counter and registers, the shelves of this fine drugstore are filled with drugs bottles and jars, patent medicines, and scales, in addition to apothecary equipment and tools, barrels and boxes of dry goods, household health supplies, quaint remedies, and big glass jars of penny candy.

KANSAS

Topeka

Kansas State Historical Society Museum
(Medico–Pharmaceutical Exhibits)
10th and Jackson Streets 66612
(913) 296-3251 / 4783
Owned and operated by the Kansas State Historical Society;
   Mark A. Hunt, museum director.

8:00 A.M. – 5:00 P.M.	Monday – Saturday
1:30 P.M. – 5:00 P.M.	Sunday

Free

There are three kinds of exhibits in the museum.
   Military medicine featuring traveling kits, dental equipment and tools

including extractors, fillings, dentures, dentifrices, and a representation of Kansas local dental practice of yesteryear.

Medical equipment and surgical instruments, medicine chests, forceps, foot doctor's equipment and utensils, Civil War period artifacts, a period room of about 1900 with examining table, devices, medical utensils, eye-examination chart, desks, certificates, stethoscopes and other examining devices, reference archival material, and tools.

Pharmaceutical equipment, tools, medicine bottles and patent medicines, drug kits, scarificators, drug jars, and pharmaceutical artifacts from the Civil War period to the turn of the century.

Study collections are accessible for interested researchers and historians.

Topeka

The Menninger Foundation Museum
P.O. Box 829
5600 West Sixth Street 66601
(913) 234-9566
Located in the tower building on the West Campus of the
    Menninger Foundation. Owned and operated by the Menninger
    Foundation, Dr. Robert Menninger, director.

8:45 A.M. – 4:30 P.M.   Monday – Friday

Free

The museum is primarily concerned with the history and practice of psychiatry as well as the Menninger family history and archives since the founding of the clinic in 1919. It includes a fine collection of Indian artifacts, pottery, jewelry, rugs, fetishes, and medicine-man masks and equipment, as well as an early Utica crib.

KENTUCKY

Danville

The McDowell House and Apothecary Shop
125-127 South Second Street 40422
(606) 236-2804
Owned and operated under the auspices of the McDowell House
    Committee of the Kentucky State Medical Association;
    George W. Grider, curator.

10 A.M. – noon and 1 P.M. – 4 P.M.   Monday – Saturday
2 P.M. – 4 P.M.   Sunday
November 1–March 1   closed Mondays, Thanksgiving,
Christmas, New Year's Day and Easter

Adults, $1.50; children under 12, 50¢.

An authentic restoration to commemorate Dr. Ephraim S. McDowell (1771-1830), the father of abdominal surgery who in 1809 was the first to successfully remove an ovarian tumor and is considered America's most famous frontier physician and surgeon. The original house, apothecary shop, and two gardens were restored through the assistance of the Kentucky State Medical Association. McDowell's apothecary shop is believed to have been the first drugstore west of the Alleghenies. In 1795, Dr. McDowell and a physician partner started medical practice together by dispensing medications in the restored two-room brick building. The front room was used as an apothecary shop continuously until 1856 while the back room was the doctor's office. The restored apothecary shop was furnished and dedicated as a

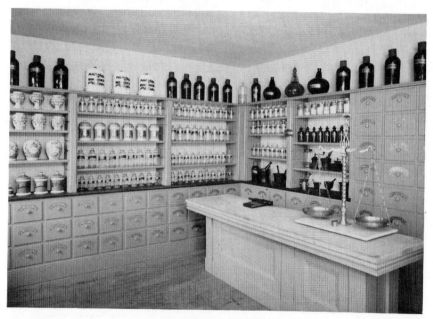

Restored interior view of what is considered to be the first apothecary shop west of the Alleghenies which was opened by the renowned surgeon, Dr. Ephraim McDowell at Danville, Kentucky in 1795. (Photo courtesy of George W. Grider, pharmacist and curator)

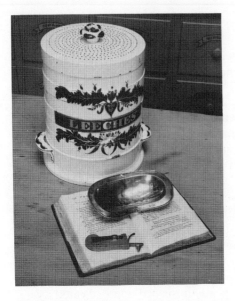

A leech jar, a bleeding bowl, a blood-letting knife, and a rare medico-pharmaceutical book are in the unusual McDowell apothecary shop at Danville, Kentucky, which was in operation from 1795 into the 1860s. (Photo courtesy of George W. Grider, pharmacist and curator)

pharmacy museum in 1959 by the Kentucky Pharmaceutical Association and aided by pharmaceutical manufacturing companies. It contains a large collection of late-eighteenth and early-nineteenth century apothecary equipment, furnishings, and utensils. These include syrups and extracts, English delft drug jars, colorful Scottish carboy-shaped stock bottles and other glassware, queensware, English leech and tobacco jars, scales (including an 1842 rare brass Austrian balance), mortars and pestles, a chest with seventy-six gold-labeled drawers with herbs, crude drugs, and chemicals.

Harrodsburg

Pleasant Hill—Shaker Village Herb Processing Exhibit
Route 4   40330
(606) 734-5411
Owned and operated by Shakertown and Pleasant Hill, Inc., and administered by a Board of Trustees.

9 A.M. – 5 P.M.   daily, mid-March through Thanksgiving weekend

Adults, $3.50; students (12–18), $1.50; children (6–11), 75¢; under age 6, free.

Shaker medicinal plants with nineteenth-century equipment and tools used in the preparation of herbs such as drying racks, pill dryers, herb cradle, herb mincer, herb press, screens, and a press for labeling products. Next to the building is an herb garden, which is included in the tour.

Richmond

Apothecary Jars Display
Eastern Kentucky University
300 Carl D. Perkins Building 40475
(606) 622-5585
Owned and operated by the Jonathan Truman Dorris Museum,
Jane E. Monson, curator. (This museum was relocated in January
1980 and does not plan to reopen until January 1985.)

8 A.M. – 4 P.M.   Monday – Friday, during regular school terms;
other times by appointment only

Free

Focusing on Kentucky's history with special emphasis on the nineteenth
century. Besides a full-scale completely furnished log cabin and spinning
and weaving demonstrations, there is a display of an 1890s collection of
apothecary jars, hospital tools, and a period library.

LOUISIANA

New Orleans

La Pharmacie Française: Historical Pharmacy Museum
514 Chartres Street 70130
(504) 586-4392
Owned and operated by the Department of Property Management
of the city of New Orleans, City Hall 70112; Pharmacist
Benjamin Bavly, honorary curator.

10 A.M. – 5 P.M.   Tuesday – Saturday

25¢

This is the original building erected by Louis Joseph Dufilho, one of
America's first licensed pharmacists, in 1823. It is in the heart of the
French Quarter (Vieux Carré). The museum was officially dedicated and
opened to the public in 1950. The ground floor portrays a mid-nineteenth century apothecary shop with pharmacy jars, decorative apothecary show globes, and specie jars on the shelves in beautiful rosewood
wall cabinets. There is a period soda fountain and an early cosmetic
case, and there are many proprietary medicines of the pre-"Pure Food
and Drug" law era in the cabinets, as well as nostrums of other periods.
Tools of the apothecary and equipment of the prescription laboratory
are displayed, as well as many medical implements. Bleeding devices
such as scarificators, fleems, and a leech jar, of the seventeenth and

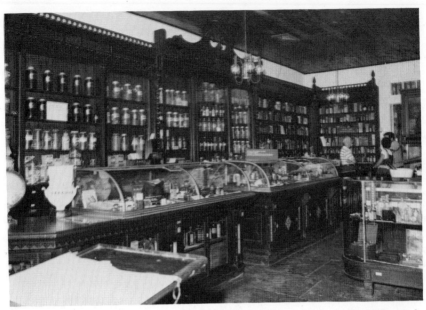

One of the finest nineteenth-century pharmacy museums in the United States is La Pharmacie Française: Historical Pharmacy Museum located in the heart of Vieux Carré at New Orleans, Louisiana.

eighteenth centuries are exhibited, along with early pharmacopeias and prescription books of a century ago, and a facsimile of a 4,000-year old cuneiform formulary.

In the rear of the apothecary is a charming old-world patio, which has been transformed into a replica of an early botanical garden. Some eighteenth-century pharmacies in Louisiana did have gardens attached.

On the second and third floors are reconstructions of mid-nineteenth-century drugstores, with invoices and ledgers dating back a century or more. The top floor has an apartment which was re-created to resemble one in which Mr. Dufilho and his family resided. There is a four-poster bed, armoire, and chairs. Another room has dining table, chairs, commode, and a marble-topped china cabinet by Mallard, a cabinetmaker of the 1850s.

For references, see David L. Cowen, "French pharmacy in Louisiana in the late 18th and early 19th centuries," *Die Vorträge der Hauptversammlung in Paris* (Stuttgart: Intern. Gesell. Gesch. Pharm., 1975), pp. 21-27.

Sabbathday Lake

Shaker's Apothecary Shop and Herb Garden
Shaker Museum 04274
(207) 926-4865
Located on Sabbathday Lake Shaker Community, Poland Spring,
on Route 26, 8 miles north of Gray (exit 11); or 12 miles south of
Auburn. Owned and operated by the United Society of Shakers;
Brother Theodore E. Johnson, director.

10:00 A.M. – 4:30 P.M.   Tuesday – Saturday, May 30 – Labor
Day, or by appointment.

Adults, $2; children under 12 years, $1; walking tour including visit
to the herb garden, $3.50.

This museum, devoted to Shaker artifacts and archives and part of a
Shaker Village was opened to the public in 1931. Presently it occupies
three buildings comprising seventeen rooms. The herb garden contains
some eighty kinds of herbs and teas from anise and dandelion to parsley
and witch hazel, which are planted, grown, harvested, dried, processed,
packed, labeled, and sold nationwide.

The apothecary shop houses an extensive collection of equipment and
tools used in drug manufacturing such as kettles, stills, presses, pill
makers, percolators, herb cutters, drying racks, grinders, and other
utensils, goods, and furnishings made or used by the Shakers. In
addition, there are extensive collections of medicine bottles, packaged
herbs and spices, posters, almanacs from about 1880, and other archival
materials and monographs.

Waterville

The La Verdiere Apothecary
Redington Museum
64 Silver Street
P.O. Box 1014   04901
(207) 873-1151
Owned and operated by the Redington Museum, The Waterville
Historical Society, and donated in its entirety by Reginald
Evariste La Verdiere, president of the La Verdiere's Super Drug
Stores; Mrs. Agatha Fullam, custodian.

2 P.M. – 6 P.M.   Tuesday – Saturday, May 15–October 1
Tours by previous arrangement

Adults, $1; children to 18, free.

The two-story wooden museum house, built in 1824, was donated by
Asa Redington's heirs to the Waterville Historical Society in 1924. The
Apothecary Annex opened in July 1976. A replica of a nineteenth-century drug store, it includes a skillfully engraved mahogany and Tiffany
soda fountain and fixtures, a phone booth, prescription ledgers dating
back to 1801, medicine and herb containers, a codfish-shape bottle
containing cod-liver oil, drug jars, show globes, show cases, posters,
period cabinets and shelving, and tools of the apothecary.

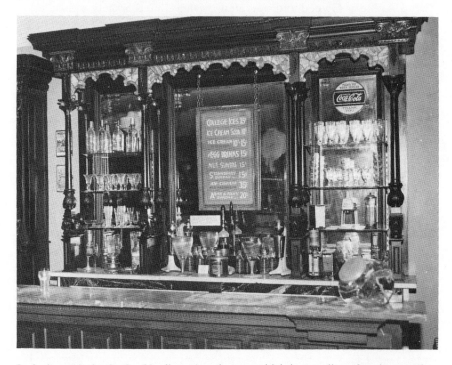

Soda fountain in the La Verdiere Apothecary which is a replica of a nineteenth-
century drugstore. It is a part of the Redington Museum in Waterville, Maine.
(Photo courtesy of La Verdiere's Super Drug Stores, Winslow, Maine)

MARYLAND

Baltimore

Cole Pharmacy Museum
E.F. Kelly Memorial Building
650 West Lombard Street 21201
(301) 727-0746
Owned and operated by the Maryland Pharmaceutical Association.

9 A.M. – 5 P.M.   Monday – Friday

Free

The museum, which opened in 1966, was named after Bessie Olive Cole —the first woman to become a professor of pharmacy administration and acting dean at the Maryland College of Pharmacy—and houses her memorabilia. It also displays pictures, prints, and archives related to pharmacist-lawyer Robert L. Swain (1887-1965), for many years editor of *Drug Topics;* and a bust of the association-executive and pharmacist-educator, E.F. Kelly (1879-1944). The museum has an extensive collection of pharmaceutical glassware, show globes, jars, patent medicines, and equipment and tools of the apothecary from the late eighteenth century to about 1900, including a seventeenth-century Spanish brass mortar, an 1805 gold coin scale by Johann Caspar, and elegant show globes.

MASSACHUSETTS

Abington

Dyer Memorial Library and Apothecary Shop
71 Center Avenue 02351
(617) 878-8480
Owned and operated by the trustees of the M.W. Dyer Memorial Library, founded in 1933; Evelyn C. Coughlan, curator.

2:30 P.M. – 5:00 P.M. and 6:30 P.M. – 8:30 P.M.   Monday, Tuesday, Thursday, Friday
Closed Sunday, Wednesday, and Saturday; other times by appointment

Free

Dedicated in 1970 "to those physicians who made their rounds on horseback and to the apothecaries who practiced the curing trade in Old Abington in the good old days." A reconstructed shop inspired in its physical design by the story of Christopher and Charles Marshall of eighteenth-century Philadelphia, as depicted in George A. Bender's *Great Moments in Pharmacy* painted by Robert Thom.

On exhibit are surgical instruments used by Drs. H.H. Dudley and Gridley Thaxter, a ship's surgeon and "physic" during the American Revolution and Thaxter's son, who practiced at Abington during the horse-and-buggy era.

On display are nineteenth-century pharmaceutical equipment and tools, patent drugs, shelf ware, medical kits and saddle bags, dried herbs, glass-labeled tincture and salt-mouth bottles, a marble-topped pan and candy scales, medical and surgical instruments, prescription registers of Drs. F.L. Bemis (1871-78), J.C. Hovey (1885-88), and C.D. Nash (1914–16), and other medico-pharmaceutical books and archival materials.

Boston

Lindemann Apothecary Collection
Massachusetts College of Pharmacy and Allied Health Sciences
    Gallery, Sheppard Library
179 Longwood Avenue 02115
(617) 732-2810
Owned and operated by the Massachusetts College of Pharmacy
    and Allied Health Sciences. Some of the collection is on display,
    but most is in storage. Apply for guided tour at the general office
    of the college.

9 A.M. – 5 P.M.   Monday – Friday, except holidays

Free

European nested weights and measures, drug jars, bottles, medicine kits, show globes, glass window displays, and pharmaceutical tools from the Joseph S. Lindemann Collection of Smith, Miller and Patch, Inc.

Brewster

Schmidt's Apothecary Shop
Route 6a   02631
(617) 896-5711
Owned and operated by the New England Fire and History
    Museum, Mrs. Joselyn N. Morris, assistant director.

10 A.M. – 5 P.M.   daily, June 15–September 15
Tours by appointment
During the winter season, write to: A. Schmidt's Apothecary,
    c/o Morris, Robert Drive, Chatham, New Jersey 07928.

Adults, $2.75; children (6–12), $1.75; under 6, free
Tour includes the entire museum

The original pharmacy was founded by pharmacist Adolph Schmidt of Germany in the late nineteenth century at Hoboken, New Jersey. It continued in operation under his nephew, Louis, until 1971.

On display in original cabinets and counters are over 1,000 matched bottles with original drugs and herbs, as well as six busts of historic alchemists, a rare "poison" closet, working bench, and pharmaceutical books and registers.

Cambridge

Botanical Museum of Harvard University
Oxford Street 02138
(617) 868-7600
Affiliated with Harvard University.

9:00 A.M. – 4:30 P.M.   Monday – Saturday
1:00 P.M. – 4:30 P.M.   Sunday
Closed on national holidays

Adults, $1.00; children, 50¢; Friday, free

Features economic botany, paleobotany, unique collection of L. and R. Blaschka glass models of plants, Hankins collection of fossil woods, a variety of crude drugs, and pharmaceutical utensils.

On 22 Divinity Avenue, there is the Gray Herbarium (telephone: 495-2364) founded at Harvard in 1864; it is devoted to botany with important specimens of flowering plants, gymnosperms, and ferns (open to students and professionals).

East Bridgewater

Dr. Hector Orr House and Apothecary Museum
The Standish Museums and First Parish Unitarian Church
The Old Common 02333
(617) 378-2467
Take Route 106 or 27.
Owned and operated by the First Parish Unitarian Church; Rev. Paul John Rich, pastor.

10 A.M. – 5 P.M.   Monday – Saturday
1 P.M. – 5 P.M.   Sunday

Adults, $1; children free. Guided tours may be arranged.

Besides an eighteenth-century church and art gallery with special exhibits which change monthly, the Standish Museums include an apothecary shop. This is a restoration of Dr. Hector Orr's 1749 house which recalls living conditions and activities of early doctors of the Plymouth Colony who made their rounds on horseback. At home, they operated a pharmacy shop where patients and clients could buy not only medicines and spices, but lottery tickets, paint, dyes, and inks. This early eighteenth-century house is probably the oldest in East Bridgewater and the original paneling and hardware are remarkably preserved. The reconstructed apothecary shop and doctor's office is a representation of the eighteenth and early-nineteenth century.

On display are drug containers and patent medicines as well as tools and equipment of the apothecary.

Northborough

Early Pharmacy Display
52 Main Street 01532
Owned and operated by Northborough Historical Society, Inc.;
    Christine L. Fipphen, curator, and Robert A. Kennerly, director.

2 P.M. – 4 P.M.   Wednesday, Saturday, May 15–September 30

Free

A pharmacy display of the late eighteenth century (opened 1961), which includes, besides regional pharmaceutical tools and objects, saddlebags, scales, and bloodletting instruments used by Stephen Ball, a physician of the Revolutionary period.

Pittsfield

Shaker's Pharmaceutical Exhibition
Hancock Shaker Community, Inc. 01201
(413) 443-0188
Located five miles west of Pittsfield, on U.S. 20. Owned and
    operated by the Shaker's Community, Inc.; Lawrence K. Miller,
    president; John H. Ott, director.

9:30 A.M. – 5:00 P.M.   daily, June 1–October 31
Winter season and groups by appointment

Adults, $3.50; children, $1.00; special rate for groups

Among twenty-one buildings, the pharmacy and herb exhibit is located in the machine-laundry shop and the brick dwelling, where several rooms are devoted to objects and equipments used in the herb and drug industry including dried herbs, old medicinal bottles prepared by the Shakers, herb packages, mortars and pestles, cutters, and drying racks. An herb garden is also included in the tour, and herb products raised and packaged in the village are available for sale.

Salem

Old New England Apothecary Shop
Historical Museum, John Ward House
132 Essex Institute 01970
(617) 744-3390
Owned and operated by the Essex Institute, Anne Farnum, curator.

10 A.M. – 4 P.M.	Tuesday – Saturday, June 1–October 15
2:00 P.M. – 4:30 P.M.	Sunday (closed Monday)

Adults, $1.00; children, 50¢

One-room reconstruction within the seventeenth-century Ward House. The authentic fixtures and furnishings came from an apothecary shop established in Salem in 1822 by Dr. William Webb. It contains tools and basic equipment of the 1830–1850 period, and is of particular local interest.

Also in the collections of the Essex Institute Museum (open all year, 9:00 A.M. – 4:30 P.M., Tuesday – Saturday; 1 P.M. – 5 P.M., Sunday; admission, $1) are other pharmaceutical items including a bust of Paracelsus (ca. 1840) from the Ennerton Apothecary Shop. They may be seen by appointment.

MICHIGAN

Alpena

Spens Drugstore Window Display
Jesse Besser Museum
491 Johnson Street 49707
(517) 356-2202
Located in the 1890s Avenue of Shops.
Owned and operated by the Jesse Besser Museum; Dennis R.
    Bodem, director.

9 A.M. – 5 P.M.	Monday – Friday
7 P.M. – 9 P.M.	Thursday
1 P.M. – 5 P.M.	Saturday, Sunday

Free; donations suggested. For Sky Theatre Planetarium: adults, $1.00; students, 50¢.
Guided tours available by appointment.

The museum was established by industrialist-benefactor Jesse Besser (1881-1970) and opened to the public in 1966. It is a regional museum illustrating growth in art, history, technology, and the natural sciences. The drugstore is a store-front window display in the museum's 1890s Avenue of Shops. The exhibit includes numerous pharmaceutical bottles, paraphernalia, and ephemera, as well as an unusual large etched-surface show globe. The drugstore is one of twelve stores on the avenue.

Dearborn

American Pharmaceutical Antiques
Oakwood Boulevard, Greenfield Village and Henry Ford Museum
   48121
(313) 271-1620
Owned and operated by Edison Institute, Inc.; Dorothy Tasker, marketing manager.

9 A.M. – 5 P.M.	daily in winter, except Thanksgiving, Christmas, and New Year's Day
9 A.M. – 6 P.M.	daily, in summer

Adults, $4.25; children (6-12), $2.25; under 6, free; special discount rates for groups are available.

This indoor-outdoor museum complex encompasses about 100 historical structures on 240 acres in Greenfield Village and the extensive Henry Ford Museum on 14 more acres (founded 1929).

Among its many exhibits are ceramic drug jars, glassware, lighting devices, domestic arts and crafts, and pharmaceutical utensils, tools, and medicine bottles.

Detroit

Early Detroit Drug Store
Detroit Historical Museum
5401 Woodward at Kirby 48202
(313) 833-1805
Owned and operated by the City of Detroit Historical Commission (Department); Solan W. Weeks, director.

9:30 A.M. – 5:00 P.M.	Tuesday, Thursday – Saturday
1 P.M. – 9 P.M.	Wednesday
1 P.M. – 5 P.M.	Sunday

Voluntary donation

The drugstore is installed on the ground floor in the "Turn of the Century Streets of Old Detroit" exhibit. It represents a simulated 1895–1905 pharmacy restoration, reflecting the "Age of Masonry." This walk-in exhibit displays artifacts and decorative embellishments collected over fifteen years. Dominating the side wall is a massive cabinet made by the Sable Store and Office Furniture Company of Detroit. The drawers are covered with protective galvanized metal, and the shelves are stocked with hand-blown and molded, glass-labeled medicinal bottles, proprietary drugs, cosmetic vases, and tin Parke, Davis and Company pressed-herb cans. Many of these drugs were salvaged from a supply house for druggists earmarked for demolition by the city as part of the Civic Center Development Project. On display also are beautifully illuminated pendant show globes filled with a period coloring formula to catch the attention of passersby, an original soda fountain complete with dispensers, soda bottles, candy and apothecary jars, and an ice-cream table and chairs.

In keeping with the period, the floor is laid with white oak, and the ceiling is paneled with authentic sculptured metal with miniature lights—donated by a local monastery—patterned after those used in commercial enterprises of the time. An original electric fan hangs from the center of the ceiling.

The plaster walls are brightened by numerous prints and patent-medicine advertisements in ironic juxtaposition beside two 1895 professional documents in rich Victorian frames. There is a pharmacy diploma from the Detroit College of Medicine, and a Michigan registered pharmacist's certificate. Installed behind the side door is one of Detroit's early gravity pull-chain water closets. In addition, the museum's collection contains 2,000 items from George A. Bender's Collection, which exemplifies the growth of Parke, Davis and Company as well as America's pharmaceutical industry as a whole.

Detroit

Pharmuseum
105 Health Sciences Building
1400 Chrysler Freeway 48202
(313) 577-1574

Owned and operated by Wayne State University's College of
Pharmacy and Allied Health Professions; Dr. Eberhard F.
Mammen, M.D., dean.

Weekdays, during school hours of the academic year or by
appointment

Free

Intended to train pharmacy students in the use of old equipment with
demonstration at a "live" display. It was donated to the college by
pharmacist Howard Mordue and other patrons.

The display consists of the "Apothecariana," comprising artifacts,
equipments and other pharmaceutical furnishings, and medicine bottles
and utensils.

Grand Rapids

DeKruif and Rudell Drug Stores Exhibition
Grand Rapids Public Museum
54 Jefferson Avenue, S.E. 45903
(616) 456-5494
Owned and operated by Grand Rapids Public Museum under the
auspices of the City of Grand Rapids; W.D. Frankforter,

10 A.M. – 5 P.M.	Monday – Friday
1 P.M. – 5 P.M.	Saturday, Sunday, and holidays; closed Christmas Day

Free

The exhibition consists of two drugstore restorations.

The J. DeKruif and Company display in the "Gaslight Village of
Shops" represents the pre-1900 era. It includes a prescription counter
with foil and painted signs for "Parke, Davis and Company's Standard
Medicinal Preparations" on the one side, and Seely's "American
Perfumery and Toilet Articles" on the other. Also on display is a soda
fountain with back bar containing stained-glass panels and an early
white ceramic Coca-Cola dispenser with gold trim.

The William Rudell Drugstore opened in August of 1900 at Sault
Sainte Marie, Michigan. It was operated by the Rudell family until it
was transported and reassembled here in August 1971 as the first of a
series of shops in the museum's "Old Town" section in the East Building. Over 15,000 items in the collection represent a complete display of
an early-1900s American pharmacy. On display are custom-built show
cases, cherry-wood wall cabinets with delicately carved garlands, and

original brass light fixtures with cut-glass shades. The prescription counter facade with Greek columns is composed of three large floor-to-ceiling mirrors separated by wooden columns with a "peep hole" in each of the center columns which enabled the practicing pharmacist to watch the store while busy behind the counter in the dispensing room. The embossed tin ceiling and circular fan are period pieces.

The shelves and drawers are filled with early proprietary remedies, herbs, and patent medicines. A dispensary, completely stocked with various drug containers and displaying original prescription records, greets the viewer who ventures into the "back shop." The floor is of colorful 1883 French ceramic tile salvaged from the old City Hall.

Manistee

The Lyman-White Drug Store
425 River Street 49660
(616) 723-5531
Owned and operated by the Manistee County Historical Society, Inc.; Steve Harold, director.

10 A.M. – 5 P.M.   Monday – Saturday
Closed Sundays and holidays, except July 4

Free

This is a restoration of the A.H. Lyman Drug Company housed from about 1880 to 1957 in a building on Manistee's main business street. It was established and operated by druggist Lyman until his death in 1904. As a wholesale drugstore, it was the first and only one in Northern Michigan above Grand Rapids. In 1904 it was purchased by Frank White, an 1891 graduate of the Philadelphia College of Pharmacy. In 1960 the building was given to the Historical Society, which devoted part of it—as well as a street show-window—to the pharmacy exhibit. It contains a large collection of intact patent-medicine packages and containers, shelf ware, and glass bottles, scales, mortars and pestles, drug grinders and sifters, pill machines, prescription files, a large collection of historical photographs, original posters, and show globes.

MINNESOTA

Grand Rapids

Trygstad Old Time Drug Store and History of Pharmacy Center, Itasca County Historical Society Museum–Central School Building

4th Street and First Avenue, N.W. 55744
(218) 326-4241 / 2418
Owned and operated by the Itasca County Historical Society;
   Dennis A. Brown, president.

9 A.M. – 5 P.M.   Monday – Saturday, May 14–October 1

Free

The collection was assembled by pharmacist Bernard H. Trygstad and exhibited in 1976 as a Bicentennial project for public view at the museum. This authentic old-time drugstore is housed in a 30×30-foot hall displaying in showcases and oak cabinets and shelves, artifacts and pharmaceutical equipment, drug jars and bottles, patent medicines, chemicals, botanicals, toiletries, and household items. Among the outstanding objects are a cachet device, an 1870 drug mill, a 1910 Eli Lilly crude-drugs identification kit, Glogau's alcohol-gas stove, a Phoenix tank dispenser, 1857 trade tokens for Holloway's pills and ointments, a collection of sixty mortars and pestles, and pharmaceutical text books.

Minneapolis

Early Pharmacy Exhibit
College of Pharmacy, University of Minnesota 55455
(612) 373-2186
Owned and operated by the University of Minnesota College of
   Pharmacy; Lawrence C. Weaver, dean.

Weekdays during school hours and by special appointment

Free

The exhibit consists of late nineteenth- and early twentieth-century American pharmacy shelf ware and tools.

South Saint Paul

Early Drug Store Exhibition
Dakota County Historical Society Museum
Municipal Building
130-3d Avenue, North 55075
(612) 451-6260
Owned and operated by the Dakota County Historical Society.

9 A.M. – 4:30 P.M.   Tuesday – Friday
9 A.M. – 1 P.M.   Saturday
Special hours and days, by appointment; conducted tours for groups
   can be arranged

Free (donations, however, are gratefully accepted).
Annual membership, $5; life membership, $50.

A small pharmacy restoration with original fixtures containing drawers for herbs and other medicines, elegant apothecary jars, patent medicines, health supplies, and other tools of the apothecary in the period of 1840–1920. Other related exhibits include a collection of surgical instruments, a fully equipped optical office, hearing aids, a medical and dental office and equipment, a barber shop, American Indian relics, agricultural products, and preserved collections of minerals, rocks, fossils, and animal and bird specimens from Dakota County.

MISSISSIPPI

University

Pharmacy Museum
School of Pharmacy–Faser Hall 38677
(601) 232-7265
Owned and operated by the University of Mississippi; Kerby E.
   Lander, Bureau of Pharmaceutical Services, director.

8:00 A.M. to 4:30 P.M.   Monday – Friday

Free

The museum opened in June 1969 at the School of Pharmacy's newly completed Faser Hall. Most of the pharmaceutical artifacts and furnishings are of late nineteenth- and early twentieth-century vintage. The general exhibit includes early prescriptions and business records, small-scale manufacturing equipment, proprietary remedies, period fixtures, a dispensing unit with etched-glass inserts, and some soda-fountain accessories.

Vicksburg

The Gerache Pharmacy Exhibition
Corner Drug Store—Corner Medical Center
1123 Washington Street 39180
(601) 636-2756
Owned and managed by pharmacist Joseph A. Gerache, proprietor,
   a 1950 graduate from the University of Loyola School of
   Pharmacy at New Orleans.

8 A.M. – 7 P.M.   Monday – Saturday

Free

A restoration of a building of the 1860s at the heart of the city's business section, purchased in 1950 and dedicated during the Bicentennial celebration on May 30, 1976. Maintaining the beauty and charm of the original structure with its Gothic style, Doric columns, high ceiling, large windows, and its geometric garden; the architecture reminds the viewer of the Civil War era when it was originally built. The collection contains period artifacts and other objects from that time and up to the early part of this century. Included are drug jars, mortars and pestles, patent medicines, show globes, medicinal bottles embossed with names of drugstores, hospitals, or name of the drug each contains, and measuring devices, weights, and scales. There are also two antique cash registers, period light fixtures, and a cast-iron gate with a mortar and pestle apothecary sign. The same building houses dental and eye clinics with artifacts.

Adjacent is the Coca-Cola Museum, originally a dry-goods store owned by H. Abraham, who sold it to the Coca-Cola Company who donated it to the City of Vicksburg for operation and maintenance. In this store, at 1107 Washington Street, the H.H. Biedenharn Candy Company bottled the first carbonated Coca-Cola sold on the market in 1894. The packages contained 6-ounce Hutchinson-stoppered bottles with the wire hook protruding from the neck when the stopper was pulled up. In 1895, a case of two dozen sold for seventy cents.

MISSOURI

Hannibal

Dr. Grant's Drug Store
Pilaster House
Southwest corner of Main and Hill Streets 63401
(314) 221-9010
Owned and operated by the City of Hannibal, Mark Twain Home
   Board, 208 Hill Street (63401); Henry Sweets, curator.

Open daily; hours vary according to season

Free

This two-story house where John M. Clemens—Mark Twain's father—died in 1847 was given to the city (1956) by Mrs. Dulany Mahan. It consists of living quarters with period fixtures and furnishings, kitchen, doctor's office, and Dr. Grant's drugstore. It contains a Fairbank iron scale and pharmacy tools, as well as patent medicines and glass containers of the second half of the nineteenth century. A decorated sign reads, "Prescriptions Accurately Compounded."

The original timbers came from Cincinnati and were brought to Hannibal in 1837 on a steamboat. The building is architecturally one of the most interesting in the city. Here, the Clemens family lived for a brief period.

Point Lookout

The Leyerle Apothecary Exhibit
Ralph Foster Museum
School of the Ozarks College 65726
(417) 334-6411, ext. 407
Located on U.S. Highway 65, 40 miles south of Springfield, Missouri; Robert S. Esworthy, director.

9 A.M. – 5 P.M.	Monday – Saturday
1 P.M. – 5 P.M.	Sunday

Free

The exhibit contains eighteenth- and nineteenth-century American and European artifacts and tools of the apothecary collected by a Springfield pharmacist, Daniel L. Leyerle, a 1910 graduate of the St. Louis College of Pharmacy. Included are early show globes; a large German-made bell-shaped mortar inscribed with the name of the artisan, Heinrich Horst, 1657; English creamware leech jar; a pair of amethyst-colored, hand-blown carboys; and a vast variety of jars, medical texts, and medicinal bottles and artifacts—in a museum that houses the finest facilities and collections in the Ozarks. The museum is also known as the "Smithsonian of the Ozarks."

St. Louis

Early Pharmacy Exhibit
St. Louis College of Pharmacy
4588 Parkview Place 63110
(314) 367-8700
Owned and operated by St. Louis College of Pharmacy; B.A. Barnes, dean.

During school hours	Monday – Friday

Free

Pharmaceutical mortars and pestles from the Max Warsaw Collection are displayed in two show windows.

St. Louis

St. Louis Medical Museum
St. Louis Medical Society Building
3839 Lindell Boulevard 63108
(314) 531-0404
Owned and operated by the St. Louis Society for Medical and
   Scientific Education; Hollister S. Smith, director.

11 A.M. – 4 P.M.   daily (closed on Sundays in winter)

Free, school tours by reservation (limit, 120 at a time)

The pharmacy collection is displayed in the nineteenth-century fixtures
from St. Vincent's Hospital in Indianapolis and Alexian Brothers Hospital in St. Louis, including a hand-carved light-oak counter with a marble
top of the 1880s. Other drug and pharmaceutical artifacts came from St.
Louis donors including the St. Louis College of Pharmacy. The museum
was founded in 1964 and accredited in 1971 by the American Association of Museums. The collection includes show globes, a prescription
counter used for dispensing drugs a century ago, suppository molds,
scales, pill tiles, and other tools of the apothecary. Also on display are
patent medicines, crude drugs and homeopathic medicines, a variety of
drug jars, mills and bottles, as well as a display of medicinal herbs drying from the rafters. The medical and dental history begins with the
works of Paracelsus and extends through Indian medicine to Doctor
Saugrain's workshop of 1800 in St. Louis to the nineteenth-century
offices of William J. Harris, M.D., and E.P. Brady, D.D.S. Their
equipment includes furnishings, medicine kits, saddle bags, portraits,
instruments, and medicine cabinets. Other sections of the museum display a large collection of X-ray devices, tubes, fluoroscopes, and stereo-
scopes. The world's oldest "transparent woman" from the 1933 Chicago
World's Fair and the Food and Drug Administration's National Museum
of Medical Quackery draw many visitors. The museum is a remarkable
exhibit of medico-pharmaceutical Americana.

MONTANA

Stevensville

Father Ravalli Pharmacy
St. Mary's Parish, Box 228   59870
(406) 777-5574
Owned and operated by the Roman Catholic Diocese of Helena;
   Most Rev. Elden F. Curtiss, Bishop.

By appointment with the pastor of St. Mary's Parish, Father James
P. Gannon
Professional guides available, May 30 – Labor Day, Hours
10 A.M. – 6 P.M.

Free

This drugstore restoration contains period fixtures, patent medicines, drawers for herbs, show globes, elegant dispensing counter, shelf ware, and pharmacy utensils from the late nineteenth century to the early 1900s.

Within the "Homes and Shops Building" exhibit, there is a doctor's office with medical tools and equipment, a barber shop, and authentic kitchens with period utensils and furnishings. Twenty-three more buildings on twenty acres show the founder's attempt since the establishment of the village in 1953 to present "a memorial to the pioneers."

NEW HAMPSHIRE

East Canterbury

Shaker's Drug Exhibition
Canterbury Shaker Museum 03224
(603) 783-9822
Located about 13½ miles northwest of Concord, on U.S. Highway 4
and Nebraska Highway 202, about four miles from the town.
Owned and operated by the Shaker Village, Inc.; J.E. Auchmoody,
executive director.

9 A.M. – 5 P.M.   Tuesday to Saturday, May 20 – October 11.
Winter season, by special appointment

Adults, $3; children $1; group rates are available, including guided
tour of the herb garden.

The herb-pharmacy exhibition is located in the Meeting House building, one of the first among twenty buildings in this Shaker village, founded in 1792. It includes herb packages, medicine bottles, vacuum pans, boxes for packaging and shipping of merchandise, pans for making syrups, rack for drying herbs, distilling apparatus, and presses.

NEW JERSEY

Absecon (town of Smithville)

Mortar and Pestle Apothecary Shop
The Old Village in the Historic Towne of Smithville
Route 9   08201
(609) 652-7777
Located 12 miles north of Atlantic City.
Owned and operated by the Historic Smithville Inns, Inc., a subsidiary of American Broadcasting Companies, Inc.; Catherine T. Hilferty, marketing administrator.

10 A.M. – 3 P.M.   Tuesday – Friday, June
10 A.M. – 5 P.M.   Tuesday – Friday, July and August
11:30 A.M. – 5:00 P.M.   Saturday – Sunday, September and October
Closed Monday

Adults, $2.50; students (5–17), $1.50; under 5, free
Special rates for groups and senior citizens

One of about thirty-seven authentic buildings relocated and restored around an historic inn founded in 1787. The restored drugstore, with its stained-glass and front windows, was originally owned by a physician-pharmacist, John Lewis Lane (Jefferson Medical College graduate, 1888) of Manahawkin, New Jersey. The authentic fixtures, apothecary jars, hand-blown glass bottles, medicine stocks, and pharmacy implements and shelf ware are from the pharmacy of Louis Segrest (graduated 1870) and William McClure (graduated 1900) of Philadelphia, which continued to about 1960.

The entire exhibition is intended to re-create a typical southern New Jersey crossroads community of the nineteenth century with typical period crafts and constructions.

Princeton

Bainbridge House
Historical Society of Princeton
158 Nassau Street 08540
(609) 921-6748 / 6817
Owned and operated by the Historical Society of Princeton; Alice O. Brown, administrator.

10 A.M. – 4 P.M.   Tuesday – Friday
2 P.M. – 4 P.M.   Saturday, Sunday
Closed Monday

Free

A restoration (completed 1970) of the original house in which William Bainbridge (U.S. Navy Commander of the *Constitution* in the War of 1812) was born in 1774. His father, Absalom Bainbridge, started his medical practice in this house. The room used as his clinic and apothecary shop is now restored with objects ranging from a pewter platter of 1762 to period furniture, bed-warming pans, bloodletting bowl, brass mortar and pestle, furnace and utensils, and nineteenth-century apothecary tools, including a pill machine, books, and prescriptions. Of interest also is a painting of Sir Hans Sloane (1660–1753), physician to King George II, by T. Murry Pinx.

In 1876, this house was purchased by the College of New Jersey (now Princeton University), which allowed it to be used as a public library (1911–66) and since 1967 made it available to the Historical Society. As a result of careful reconstruction, it is an excellent example of eighteenth-century architecture, as well as exemplifying the office of a physician-pharmacist of the period.

NEW MEXICO

Albuquerque

Pharmacy Museum
College of Pharmacy, The University of New Mexico 87131
(505) 277-2461
Owned and operated by the University of New Mexico College of
  Pharmacy; Carman A. Bliss, dean.

By arrangement with the dean's office

Free

The museum has a prescription counter and showcases with pharmaceutical artifacts from about the turn of the century. The emphasis is on local and regional history including the history of the college. On display also are objects related to folklore therapeutic agents, especially of southwest Spanish and Indian medicinal herbs and "cures."

NEW YORK

Albany

Throop Drug Store Restoration
Albany College of Pharmacy
Union University

106 New Scotland Avenue 12208
(518) 445-7211 / 7253
Owned and operated by the college; Walter Singer, dean.

9 A.M. – 4 P.M.   Monday – Friday

Free

This is an authentic restoration of the Jabez W. Throop drugstore of
Schoharie, 40 miles from the New York state capital. Established in
1800, it continued operation at the same location and in the same family
until 1936. It was thereafter moved intact to the College of Pharmacy as
an historical museum. Its original fixtures reflect a rural American pharmacy shop a century ago. The stove, the kerosene oil lamp, the waste-
paper container, the ball of twine, the cuspidor, the show globes, and
the wooden safe—covered with iron sheeting and knobs—are all period
pieces. The fixtures of pine wood have scrollwork, hand-carved
brackets, and labeled drawers with porcelain pulls where herbs and
medicines were stored. Other items include patent medicines, circulars,
posters, pharmacy registers, glass bottles, artificial nipples, and a period
microscope.

Brooklyn

Pharmaceutical Show Cases
Arnold and Marie Schwartz College of Pharmacy and Health
    Sciences
75 DeKalb Avenue at University Plaza 11201
(212) 330-2700
Owned and operated by the college, Long Island University, John
    J. Sciarra, dean.

9 A.M. – 5 P.M.   Monday – Friday

Free

Exhibit cases installed in the lobby display pharmaceutical tools, glass
bottles, patent medicines, and other pharmacy-related memorabilia.

Brooklyn

Pharmacy Exhibition
· The Brooklyn Museum
188 Eastern Parkway 11238
(212) 638-5000
Owned and operated by the Brooklyn Museum's Department of
    Decorative Arts.

10 A.M. – 5 P.M.	Wednesday – Saturday	
12 noon – 5 P.M.	Sunday; 1 P.M. – 5 P.M.	holidays
Closed Monday, Tuesday, and Christmas Day		

Free

There is a collection of ten drug pots of tin-glazed earthenware, six from Italy and four from Holland, dating from the sixteenth to the eighteenth centuries.

Buffalo

Diehl–Riggs Pharmacy Exhibit
25 Nottingham Court 14216
(716) 873-9644
Owned and operated by the Buffalo and Erie County Historical
  Society; Robert L. Damm, director.

10 A.M. – 5 P.M.	Monday – Friday
Noon – 5 P.M.	Saturday, Sunday

Free

On exhibit is an 1881 prescription unit from a pharmacy owned by C. Lewis Diehl (1840–1917), a well-known German-born American pharmacist and educator. It includes apothecary tools and artifacts, and patent medicines from the turn of the century. To these are added period pharmaceutical objects from the drugstore of C.N. Riggs, a native of Buffalo. They include a decorative marble soda-fountain unit that "enshrines eight delicious flavors," including sarsaparilla. Other objects include chemicals, drug jars and bottles, apothecary tools and sundries, sickroom supplies, perfumery, extracts, surgical appliances, and signs and posters, including one reading "Best pure drugs of standard strength."

Clinton

The Wagoner Apothecary Shop—Clinton Pharmaceutical Company
Park Row Pharmacy No. 77
3 West Park Row 13323
(315) 853-5529
Located 8 miles south of Utica, on Route 12 B; main entrance is
  from the present Park Row Pharmacy. Owned and operated by
  the Adam Drug Company, 75 Sabin Street, Pawtucket, Rhode
  Island 02860; Fred Brundige, pharmacist–manager.

9 A.M. – 9 P.M.	Monday – Friday
9 A.M. – 8 P.M.	Saturday
9 A.M. – 4 P.M.	Sunday

Free

This is a restoration of an apothecary shop of the late nineteenth century in the basement of the original building where the Clinton Pharmaceutical Company (presently the Bristol Myers Company) originated. It displays authentic period fixtures, desk, plank floor, drawers, and furnishings with an assortment of patent medicines, glass bottles, show globes, and tools of the apothecary. It was opened to the public in 1965 through the efforts of the late proprietor, Robert Wagoner.

Cooper

Druggist's Shop
Lake Road–Coopertown Museums 13326
(607) 547-2533
Owned and operated by the New York State Historical Association;
  Maria Zamelis, public relations.

9 A.M. – 5 P.M.	Daily, May – October
9 A.M. – 5 P.M.	Tuesday – Saturday, November – April
1 P.M. – 5 P.M.	Sunday

Closed Thanksgiving, Christmas, and New Year's Day

Adults, $3; juniors (7–15), $1.25—including the Farmer's Museum and the Fenimore House: adults $5; juniors $2

The Farmer's Museum and its village crossroads together with the Fenimore House reflect the life of ordinary people of the late eighteenth to the late nineteenth centuries.

Among a dozen restored buildings are included a country store (1820), printing office (1829), homestead barn (1796), schoolhouse (1810), and a druggist's shop from about 1832. It sold herbal medicines, perfumes, paints, and other sundries. The original fixtures come from Hartwick, New York. Adjacent to it is a doctor's office restored to about 1829, originally from Westford, New York.

Corning

Corning Pharmaceutical Glass Collection
The Corning Museum of Glass and Corning Glass Center,
Museum Way 14830
(607) 937-5371 or 974-8271

The Glass Center is affiliated with and operated by the Corning Glass Works. Founded 1951. John P. Fox, director, Glass Center; Thomas S. Buechner, director, The Corning Museum of Glass; and Clare Bavis, Visitor/Community Information, Glass Center.

9 A.M. – 5 P.M.   daily
Closed Thanksgiving, Christmas, and New Year's Day

Adults, $2

A museum of glass, its manufacturing, technology, and uses with audio-visual presentations. Among the numerous glass exhibits is a collection of medicinal glass bottles, patent medicines, and glass vases for drugs.

Monroe

Vernon Apothecary Shop
Museum Village in Orange County
Route 17   10950
(914) 782-8247
Located 1 mile west of Monroe on routes 6, 17, and 17M; 4 miles from the New York Thruway, exit 16, at Harriman. Operated by an eighteen-member Board of Trustees as a nonprofit educational institution founded in 1950 as an Old Museum Village of Smith's Clove; Jean MacDonald, public relations.

10 A.M. – 5 P.M.   daily, May 1 – October 31

Adults, $3.50; juniors (6–15 years), $2.75; group rates by reservation only.

"A treasury of 19th-century Americana." This museum village in Orange County contains thirty restored buildings and a natural history museum. The apothecary shop displays patent medicines of all sorts, a soda fountain, shelf ware, tools, and period fixtures.

New York City

Drug Jars Display
The Hispanic Society of America
155th Street and Broadway 10032
(212) 926-2234
Owned and operated by The Hispanic Society of America (founded 1904); Priscilla E. Muller, curator of the museum.

10:00 A.M. – 4:30 P.M.   Tuesday – Saturday
1 P.M. – 4 P.M.   Sunday

Closed Christmas week and first week of new year (two consecutive weeks); February 12, 22; Good Friday; Easter Sunday; May 30; July 4; October 12; and Thanksgiving weekend.

Free

Displayed is a collection of Hispano-Moresque and Talavera drug jars, one of the finest of its kind in this country.

New York City

Italian Majolica
The Metropolitan Museum of Art
Fifth Avenue at 82d Street 10028
(212) TR9-5500
Owned and operated by the museum, Jessie McNab, associate
  curator.

10:00 A.M. to 4:45 P.M.	Wednesday – Saturday
10:00 A.M. to 8:45 P.M.	Tuesday
11:00 A.M. to 4:45 P.M.	Sundays and holidays
Closed Mondays	

Adults, $2.50 suggested or any reasonable donation.

A representative collection of Italian Renaissance Majolica among which are a number of apothecary jars with the name of the drug inscribed on many of them in Latin, plus a few French sixteenth- and seventeenth- and Dutch eighteenth-century pieces. Important examples of Hispano-Moresque and other European apothecary jars and weights and measures are also on display.

On display at the Cloisters of the Metropolitan Museum of Art, Fort Tyron Park, New York City 10040, is another collection of several fine albarellos, examples of Hispano-Moresque lusterware, plates, and deep dishes, principally in the Spanish Room. For hours and admission see above.

Inquiries to see drug pots not on exhibition may be made by letter or telephone.

New York City

Lascoff Pharmaceutical Antiques Collection
The Gustave L. and Janet W. Levy Library
The Mount Sinai Medical Center
Fifth Avenue and 100th Street 10029
(212) 650-6671
Owned and operated by the Mount Sinai Medical Center's Levy
  Library; Jane S. Port, director.

By appointment

Free

The collection consists of twenty-five objects displayed in five cases, given to the Medical Center by Emma Lascoff in memory of her husband, J. Leon Lascoff. Included in the display are a large nineteenth-century counterbalance; six mortars and pestles of iron, bronze, porcelain and wood, ranging from the eighteenth through the twentieth centuries; a porcelain leech jar; and a "species diureticae" Imari jar.

New York City

Nineteenth-century Pharmacy
Chandler Museum, Department of Chemistry, 3rd floor
Havemeyer Hall, Columbia University 10027
(212) 280-2176
Owned and operated by the Department of Chemistry, Columbia
    University; Frances Hoffman, director of chemical laboratories.

9 A.M. – 5 P.M.   Monday – Friday

Free

Reconstructed nineteenth-century apothecary shop with fixtures and extensive collection of period artifacts such as shelf ware, patent medicines, and American and European drug jars and utensils. It also included chemicals and apparatus such as those prepared and used by Priestley, Lavoisier, and Harold Urey.

New York City

Pharmacy and Health Exhibits
The American Museum of Natural History
79th Street and Central Park West 10024
(212) 873-1300
Affiliated with the City University of New York and Columbia
    University and governed by a Board of Trustees.

10:00 A.M. – 4:45 P.M.   Monday – Saturday
11 A.M. – 5 P.M.   Sunday and holidays
Closed Thanksgiving and Christmas.

Free; donations accepted

The museum, founded in 1869, contains a hall on human biology, perception, health care, as well as exhibits on mineralogy, fossils, and many aspects of traditional cultures including health care.

Old Chatham

Medicine Room
The Shaker Museum Foundation, Inc.,
Shaker Museum Road 12136
(518) 794-9100
Located 5 miles from exit B-2 of the Berkshire spur of the New
York Thruway; 17 miles from Albany on U.S. 20, then south on
Route 66 and follow signs.
Owned and operated by the Shaker Museum Foundation, Inc.;
Peter Laskovski, director, and Mrs. Claire L. Wheeler, admin-
istrative assistant.

10:00 A.M. – 5:30 P.M.   daily, May 1 – October 31
Winter season, by appointment

Adults, $2.50; children (6–14), 75¢; senior citizens, $2.00; students
(15–21), $1.50

Among the thirty-six galleries is a medicine manufacturing room dup-
licating a similar room of the "First Family's Medicine Shop" at Mt.
Lebanon, New York. Much of the equipment comes from the original
shop. The dried-herb cabinet, with its four paneled doors, is a good
example of Shaker interior architectural design. On display are a work-
bench, power-driven mixing vat, a seed box, label-printing press, label-
sorting cabinet, Canterbury iron mortar and pestle, a copper alembic
used in the production of witch hazel, stoneware jugs and jars for
storage of medicinal products, and other fixtures built by the Shakers.
An herb garden is adjacent to the building and is included in the tour.

Rochester

Pierson–Benham Apothecary Hall Exhibition
Rochester Museum and Science Center
657 East Avenue 14607
(716) 271-4320
Owned by the Rochester Museum and Science Center, P.O. Box
1480 14603; Fred H. Rollins, curator.

9 A.M. – 5 P.M.   Monday – Saturday
1 P.M. – 5 P.M.   Sunday
Closed Christmas Day

Adults, $1.00; senior citizens and children, 50¢

A reconstruction of authentic shelves and drawers from the William
Pierson drugstore (founded at Canandaigua, New York, in 1830) and
continued through partnership with La Roy Benham. The fixtures were

installed in 1943 and over the years many artifacts dating from 1860-1910 were added to round out the exhibition. Included are patent medicines (especially made in the Rochester area), glassware, herbs, grinders, laboratory sink, pitcher pump, show globes, leech and tobacco jars, phrenology head, cosmetics, filters, hearing aids, nursing bottles, eyeglasses, pill rollers, splints, scales, mortars and pestles, clock showcases, decanters, and a kerosene lamp.

NORTH CAROLINA

Bailey

The Country Doctor Museum
P.O. Box 34   27807
(919) 235-4165 / 3873
Owned and operated by the Country Doctor Museum Foundation
  and ruled by a Board of Directors.

2 P.M. – 5 P.M.   Sunday, Wednesday
Closed December – February
Special groups by appointment

Free

Dedicated in 1968 in commemoration of the family doctor. This museum consists of two office reconstructions: the first built in 1857 by Dr. Howard F. Freeman, which includes an apothecary shop with period patent medicines, jars, tools, and equipment; and the second built about 1889 by Dr. Cornelius H. Brantley for his practice. This authentic composite contains a unique collection of medical memorabilia and instruments, as well as a completely furnished apothecary shop with antiques dating from the twelfth to the present century. Specific emphasis is on portraying nineteenth-century doctor-pharmacist activities in this country. An herb garden is adjacent to the museum.

Chapel Hill

Booker's Old Time Drug Exhibition
Patterson's Mill Country Store
Durham County, Route 6, Farrington Road 27514
(919) 544-2047
Located in the vicinity of the University of North Carolina. Owned
  and operated by John and Elsie Booker.

8:30 A.M. – 5:30 P.M.   Monday – Saturday
1:30 P.M. – 5:30 P.M.   Sunday

Free

One part of this general country store is devoted to a reconstructed apothecary shop with original counters, shelving, tin herb containers, tools, patent medicines, showcases, a stove, and a variety of posters from "For Constipation—LAX" and "Indian Root Pills" to "Bromo-Seltzer for Headache" and "Humphrey's Remedies." Most of the fixtures and artifacts date from about 1900 and include an old-time telephone and register, prescription cabinet and files, scales, cork pressers, "Proctor and Gamble Electric Time," Humphrey's Witch Hazel Ointment Compound for Piles, malted milk, and Munyon's Homeopathic remedies.

In addition, there is a complete doctor's office containing surgical instruments, examination chart, bed and mattress, and an 1844 cost-of-living list and doctor's fees. There are also two dental chairs and medico-pharmaceutical herbs and formularies collected over a period of more than thirty years.

Chapel Hill

Pharmacy Museum
School of Pharmacy
University of North Carolina 27514
(919) 966-1121
Owned and operated by the University of North Carolina School of
    Pharmacy; T.S. Miya, dean.

Open during school hours

Free

There are several exhibit cases with glass-labeled stock bottles, patent medicines, show globes, scales, mortars, jars, presses, and other tools of the apothecary. The museum was started in 1932 by J.G. Beard, then dean of the school.

Greensboro

Dr. William "Clark" Porter's Drugstore
(W.C. Porter and Company)
Greensboro Historical Museum
Richardson Civic Center
130 Summit Avenue 27401
(919) 373-2043
Owned and operated by the Greensboro Historical Museum, Inc.
    (founded 1924); William J. Moore, director.

10 A.M. – 5 P.M.	Tuesday – Saturday
2 P.M. – 5 P.M.	Sunday

Free

The reconstruction was dedicated as a memorial to pharmacist William Sydney Porter (1862–1910), better known as O. Henry. Here in his hometown, Porter completed his apprenticeship (1879–81) under the supervision of his uncle, Clark Porter, the pharmacy's owner. The young pharmacist later became a distinguished author. This exhibit includes some of the original fixtures and equipment used in the drugstore, as well as personal memorabilia of O. Henry and his family which are displayed in cases near the drugstore exhibit.

The Porter Drugstore exhibit is also a memorial to Lunsford Richardson, founder of Vick Chemical Company which is known today as Richardson–Merrell. Mr. Richardson bought the Elm Street drugstore from Clark Porter in 1890 and developed an ointment now known as Vicks Vaporub while working there. In 1898 he sold his retail business and established the L. Richardson Drug Company, a wholesale house which provided a wider sale for his remedies. In 1905 Mr. Richardson sold that business and established Vicks Chemical Remedies.

NORTH DAKOTA

Jamestown

Medico-Pharmaceutical Exhibit
321 Third Avenue, N.E.
P.O. Box 1002   58401
(701) 252-6741
Owned and operated by the Stutsman County Memorial Museum, affiliated with the Fort Seward Historical Society, Inc.; David J. Robertson, curator.

2 P.M. – 9 P.M.   Wednesday and Sunday, June through October
Other times by appointment

Free

On display are Indian artifacts, and medico-pharmaceutical equipment and instruments, as well as medicine bottles and tools of the apothecary.

West Fargo

Prairie Pioneer Drug Store
Bonanzaville, U.S.A.

P.O. Box 719   58078
(701) 282-2822
Located on U.S. Highway 10, 5 miles from Fargo and 1 mile west
of West Fargo. Owned and operated by the Cass County Historical Society; Mrs. Richard Carlson, curator, The Red River
and Northern Plains Regional Museum.

9:30 A.M. – 5:00 P.M.	Monday – Friday, June 1 – October 31
1:00 P.M. – 5:00 P.M.	Saturday, Sunday, June 1 – October 31
9:30 A.M. – 4:00 P.M.	Tuesday – Friday, during winter season

Adults, $2; children (6–16), $1; under 6, free.

A replica of a pioneer village, including twenty-five authentic buildings,
a drugstore restoration with original fixtures, equipment and tools from
an early 1900s drugstore in Gilby, North Dakota. It includes patent
medicines, mortars and pestles, show globes, razors, collar buttons, and
other artifacts, and pharmaceutical books and formularies. The restored
building and artifacts were secured through the generosity and efforts of
pharmacist David Olson.

OHIO

Cleveland

Cleveland Health Education Museum
8911 Euclid Avenue 44106
(216) 231-5010
Owned and operated by the Cleveland Health Education Museum;
Lowell F. Bernard, director.

9:00 A.M. – 4:30 P.M.	Monday – Saturday
1:00 P.M. – 4:30 P.M.	Sunday
Closed Thanksgiving, Christmas, and New Year's Day	

Adults, $1.50; juniors (6–18), 75¢; children under 6, free; free to
individuals on Tuesday afternoons.

Exhibits related to pharmaceutical history and education include three
permanent major displays produced by the Upjohn Company: the
Chromosome, the Brain, and the Inflammatory Process. These and
other exhibits on medicine and health attempt to present the latest
information on the systems of the human anatomy, physiology, and
human ecology. The museum staff provides health programs to children
during the school year. In thirteen experimental teaching theaters, a
wide variety of health topics is introduced in depth through the multi-

media approach. Selected exhibits trace the historical perspectives and relevance of health knowledge. This pioneer health museum which was founded in 1936 and opened in 1940 has aided in the development of similar museums in the United States and other countries. It was initiated by the local Academy of Medicine and the Dental Society under the praiseworthy efforts of its first director, Bruno Gebhard, M.D., who retired in 1956. In 1970 it developed the health-education program to provide a focal point not only for student teaching, but continued in-service teacher training, as well as providing a community resource center in health-education material. Through the newly created Multi-Media Materials Production Department, the museum is capable of preparing all of its own program materials and descriptive literature to supplement its exhibitions, and to sell to other organizations undertaking similar programs. Other exhibits of special atraction are those on brain function, nervous system, eyes and ears, the five senses, growth and development, wonder and defense of new life, microbes, and a "children health fair."

The educational department also offers courses for preschool through college grades in body systems, nutrition, dental care, drugs, environment, heredity, sexuality, and family and career planning.

Cleveland

The Dittrick Museum and Pharmaceutical Collections
The Howard Dittrick Museum of Historical Medicine
The Cleveland Medical Library Association
11000 Euclid Avenue 44106
(216) 368-3648
Owned and operated by the Cleveland Medical Library Association;
  P.A. Gerstner, chief curator.

10 A.M. – 5 P.M.	Monday – Friday, September – May
1 P.M. – 5 P.M.	Sunday, September – May
1 P.M. – 5 P.M.	Saturday, June – August; closed Sunday

Free
For guided tours, inquire about charges

This is primarily a medical museum, but contains several outstanding collections of pharmaceutical antiques and related objects. It includes drawers and shelving from the Sterniki pharmacy of about 1866, equipment from the Smithknight pharmacy (founded 1857), ointment jars from the Petersilge pharmacy (founded 1881) and other equipment from early Cleveland drugstores. Also on display are European drug jars, early microscopes, pharmacy bottles, and materials related to general hygiene. The themes featured include a visit to the doctor, X-rays, sphygmomanometers, electrocardiography, stethoscopes, hematology, urinalysis, tongue depressors, and ophthalmoscopes. Also recommended is a visit to the historical and periodicals sections of the Allen Memorial Library, home of the Cleveland Medical Library, in the same building.

Columbus

Drug Store Replica
The Durell Street of Yesteryear
Center of Science and Industry
280 East Broad Street 43215
(614) 228-6361
Owned and operated by the Center of Science and Industry.

10 A.M. – 5 P.M.	Monday – Saturday
1 P.M. – 5:30 P.M.	Sunday

Adults, $2.50; students, $1.50

This street of restored shops includes an 1865 replica of an American drugstore with authentic fixtures, shelf ware, and tools of the apothecary, sponsored by the Academy of Pharmacy of Central Ohio and the Women's Pharmacy Club.

Hillsboro

Edward B. Ayres Drug Store
114 E. Main Street 45133
(513) 393-1814
Owned and operated by the Vernon Farrley Hardwares Co.;
    pharmacist Frank O. Granger, manager.

9 A.M. – 6 P.M.	Monday, Tuesday, Thursday, Saturday
1 P.M. – 6 P.M.	Wednesday

Free

The original building was built in 1808 with the sign of the big red mortar and pestle (British made, nineteenth century). The fixtures are authentic. The shelves and cabinets are filled with old glass bottles, patent medicines, herb and tea packages, and tools of the apothecary.

Lebanon

The Golden Mortar Drug Store
105 South Broadway
P.O. Box 223   45036

(513) 932-1817
Located two doors south of the Golden Lamb Inn, Ohio's oldest hostelry, corner of State Highway 63 and U.S. Highway 42. Owned and operated by the Warren County Historical Society Museum; Elva R. Adams, director.

9 A.M. – 4 P.M.	Tuesday – Saturday
Noon – 4 P.M.	Sunday
Closed Mondays and national holidays	

Adults, $1.00; students, 25¢

This museum on local history and early artifacts from southwestern Ohio houses an extensive collection of early pharmaceutical fixtures, shelf ware, patent medicines, herbs, pharmaceutical tools, an 1856 counter, certificates, prescriptions, and filing cabinets.

New Vienna

Noble-Blackburn Drug Store
The New Vienna Pharmacy
153 Main Street 45159
(513) 987-2212
S. Roger and Luella Blackburn, proprietors–pharmacists.

9 A.M. – 6 P.M.	Monday, Tuesday, Thursday, Friday
9 A.M. – 5 P.M.	Wednesday, Saturday
Closed on Sunday	

Free

Established by W.A. Henry on January 2, 1882, it was operated by him as a pharmacy and jewelry store. The following is a list of owner–pharmacists through the following years until it was bought by the present owners, pharmacists Mr. and Mrs. Blackburn: W.A. Henry, 1882–1892; James R. West, 1892–1909; W.C. Higley, 1909–1928; and N.C. Noble, 1924–1967.

The store was operated by Mr. Noble and his heirs until it was purchased by the present owners. It includes the old cabinets and fixtures. Most of the show cases have the original glass in them. There are pharmaceutical vessels, glass-stoppered and glass-labeled storage bottles, patent medicines, glassware, drug jars, tools of the apothecary, and a soda fountain with accessories.

OKLAHOMA

Lawton

Medico-Pharmaceutical Exhibition
Museum of the Great Plains
Corner of Sixth and Ferris Streets (at Elmer Thomas Park)
P.O. Box 68   73502
(405) 353-5675
Owned and operated by the Museum and Institute of the Great
    Plains; Towana Spivey, curator of anthropology.

8 A.M. – 5 P.M.   Monday – Friday
10 A.M. – 5 P.M.   Saturday
1:30 P.M. – 5 P.M.   Sunday
Closed Thanksgiving, Christmas, and New Year's Day

Free

Within the turn-of-the-century frontier town, there is a general store
with shelves of patent medicine bottles and also a doctor-dentist-phar-
macist's office with medical instruments, a dental chair and equipment,
drug containers, and tools of the apothecary. There is also a good
collection of Indian artifacts related to the medicine man including
bundles of sacred herbs, fetishes, and other curing aids.

Oklahoma City

Dorrance Pharmacy Museum
600 N.E. Fifteenth Street 73190
(405) 271-6484
Owned and operated by the University of Oklahoma College of
    Pharmacy, 644 N.E. Fourteenth Street; Rita Pierce, curator.

8 A.M. – 5 P.M.   Monday – Friday

Free

The entire exhibition is dedicated to the memory of Lemuel Dorrance,
the first graduate pharmacist from the Department of Pharmaceutical
Chemistry in 1896—the precursor to the present University of Oklahoma College of Pharmacy. It was moved from Norman to the university's Oklahoma City Health Sciences Center in 1977. The museum displays equipment and tools of the apothecary, drug containers, patent
medicines, and fixtures dating from the 1880s to the 1950s.

OREGON

Jacksonville

Pharmaceutical Exhibit
Jacksonville Museum
206 North Fifth Street 97530
(503) 899-1847
Owned and operated by the Jackson County Historical Society; C. William Burk, director.

9 A.M. – 5 P.M.	Tuesday – Saturday
Noon – 5 P.M.	Sunday

Free

Founded in 1950, this museum contains a medico-pharmaceutical exhibit with artifacts and tools of the apothecary as well as glassware and patent medicines.

PENNSYLVANIA

Bethlehem

The Apothecary Museum
Moravian Museum of Bethlehem
Gemein Haus, 66 West Church Street 18018
(215) 867-0173
Located at rear of 420 Main Street. Owned by the Moravian Congregation of Bethlehem; shown and managed by the Moravian Museum of Bethlehem.

1 P.M. – 4 P.M.   Saturdays, April – September
Individual and group tours by appointment

Adults, 50¢; children, free

Original eighteenth-century fireplace (1752) with equipment and utensils for alchemy laboratory including retorts, grinders, and scales, as well as Delft jars, glassware, and tools of the apothecary. Adjacent is an herb and flower garden of special interest.

Doylestown

Pharmacy and Medical Antiques Study Collection
The Mercer Museum
Pine and Ashland Streets 18901

(215) 345-0210
Owned and operated by the Bucks County Historical Society.

10 A.M. – 5 P.M.	Tuesday – Saturday, March – December
1 P.M. – 5 P.M.	Sunday, March – December

Closed, January and February, Thanksgiving, and Christmas
Pharmaceutical and medical collections may be seen by
appointment.

Adults, $2.00; students, $1.00; families, $3.50
Group rates available

Henry Chapman Mercer's (1856–1930) comprehensive collection of
American antiques is assembled here. Included are pharmaceutical and
medical equipment study collections: medicinal herbs, patent medicines,
tools of the apothecary, and dental, surgical, and veterinary implements.
This is part of a general museum in which over forty early American
crafts are exhibited.

Philadelphia

Anatomical and Health Exhibition
The Wistar Institute
36th Street at Spruce 19104
(215) 243-3708
Independent nonprofit organization affiliated with the University of
Pennsylvania Medical School.

10 A.M. – 4 P.M.   Monday – Friday

Free

A memorial for Philadelphian anatomist-surgeon Caspar Wistar (1761–
1818) who served after William Shippen as the University of Pennsylvania's professor of anatomy. Incorporated in 1892, this is the first
independent biomedical institute in the United States.

On display are models, and anatomical and pathological specimens
used for teaching purposes, as well as surgical instruments, microscopes,
and rare books. Themes represented include biology, therapy, compara-
tive anatomy, heredity, and optics.

Philadelphia

Kendig Memorial Museum
Temple University Health Science Center
Fourth Floor, Room 409
3307 North Broad Street 19140
(215) 221-4956
Owned and operated by the Temple University School of

Pharmacy; John A. Lynch, curator.

During regular school hours

Free

The museum is dedicated to the memory of Dean H. Evert Kendig who served the school for over forty-two years, until his retirement in 1950. It houses a notable collection of Old World and American pharmaceutical equipment, shelf ware, specie jars, show globes, nursing bottles, mortars and pestles, and other tools of the apothecary. It was open in 1957 and moved to the new Health Sciences Center in 1974. At the entrance the visitor is greeted by two rare gaslight mortar and pestle lamp signs which are studded with gemlike crystals and flank the door to the museum.

The authentic fixtures include an elaborately carved walnut counter and matching shelves, once part of a nineteenth-century Philadelphian drugstore. The fixtures were originally housed in The Old Morgan Pharmacy at Fourteenth (Seventeenth at the time) and Walnut streets where the Wyeth Brothers—founders of the Wyeth Laboratories—had started and were donated by Irwin Kauffman.

The oldest item in the museum is an Italian brass mortar and pestle of about 1567. Of American artifacts, the earliest are two eighteenth-century glass bottles excavated near Independence Hall.

The museum houses a good collection of powder and liquid glass and ceramic drug jars, spitoon cups, and a wooden jar owned by pharmacist Christopher Sower about 1735. Other drug containers are elaborately decorated with pictures and coats of arms. One rhubarb blown-glass jar is over two feet high resembling a fancy umbrella stand. Among the technical artifacts are syringes, clysters, strainers, inhalers, powder folders, tablet machines, and ointment jars.

Philadelphia

Museum and Pharmaceutical Exhibits
The Philadelphia College of Pharmacy and Science
43d Street and Kingsessing Avenue 19104
(215) 386-5800
Located in University City Mall. Owned and operated by The Philadelphia College of Pharmacy and Science; Dr. Ara H. Der Marderosian, curator.

Weekdays during school hours

Free

Exhibits at this first school of pharmacy in the country—founded in 1821—consist of the following displays.

A general pharmacy museum in Griffith Hall includes the collections of Dr. David Costelo (Philadelphia College of Pharmacy and Science, class of 1874), Wilson McNeary (class of 1907), and Harry Darr (class of 1909). It is made up of original fixtures, old books, ornate and beautifully inscribed drug and leech jars and vessels, decorative mortars, and apothecary tools and equipment from the Old and New Worlds going back to the European Renaissance period and earlier. There are show globes, pill tiles, toilet-article signs, and an American eagle show jar with twenty-star states. The east wall of the foyer of Griffith Hall is covered with six elegant murals in oil done by William Matthews of New York, which depict various phases in the development of pharmacy from dawn of time to the present.

The George Glenworth Pharmacy shop was originally opened in 1812 on 817 Sassafras (now Race) Street on the corner of Chester in "The City of Brotherly Love." Pharmacist Glenworth was one of the founders of the college, and his shop remained in the family until 1905. On display, although partially damaged, is the only copy in existence of a "membership certificate" in the "Philadelphia College of Apothecaries" which was formed on the same lines and principles as its predecessor in London, England. Also shown are post-Civil War period fixtures and shelf ware, including drug jars, prescriptions, and archival material.

The Bohlander Drugstore includes paintings of natural scenes, pictures of medicinal plants, advertising signs and posters. There are tools of the apothecary, including suppository molds, pill tiles, mortars and pestles, and cork presses. Also on exhibit are patent medicines, microscopes, a cash register, typewriters, opium scales, a hand twiller, and drug stocks. This exhibition in Blanch Gardner Whitecar Hall is named after pharmacist George Bohlander who donated it to the college in 1975. The fixtures were made by a German-born carpenter, M.A. Heiman of Altamont, Illinois, who also designed the pharmacy fixtures and showcases including the tinted lead-glass windows. Artifacts and patent medicines were donated during 1975–78 by Benjamin Greenbaum (class of 1938), Morris Blatman (class of 1941) and Herbert Brennan (class of 1938).

The Joseph Enland Library of the college houses several collections of various pharmaceutical wares including numerous oil paintings. One is the portrait of William Proctor, the father of American pharmacy, which was donated to the college by Wyeth Laboratories.

Philadelphia

The Mütter Museum
19 South 22d Street 19103
(215) 561-6050, ext. 41

Owned and operated by the College of Physicians of Philadelphia, the oldest American private medical society in the United States, (founded 1787); Gretchen Worden, acting curator of the museum.

10 A.M. – 4 P.M. Tuesday – Friday	
Guided tours on request	

Free

The museum collection was founded in 1849 as a teaching tool in the study of disease and injury. It took formal shape during the Civil War through the financial and museum collection bequest of Dr. Thomas Dent Mütter. In 1909 it moved to its new Georgian-style home at its present address.

The museum houses a large and impressive collection of pathological specimens as well as medico-pharmaceutical artifacts and medical lore ranging from seventh-century B.C. Assyrian prescription tablets and ancient Roman surgical instruments to twentieth-century hearing aids and electrocardiographs. Other artifacts and curios include apothecary jars, patent remedies, medicine bags and kits (including those used by William Shippen and Benjamin Rush in the late eighteenth century). There are bleeding and cupping utensils, apothecary tools (scales, weights and measures, mortars and pestles, and pill tiles), papboats and nursing bottles. Also on display are X-ray tubes, obstetrical forceps and other instruments, stethoscopes, inhalers, percussion hammers, a good collection of microscopes, syringes, ophthalmoscopes, thermometers (one used by Dr. William Cullen of Edinburgh, mid-eighteenth century), spectacles, hearing aids, and surgical instruments. Walls in major halls of the college are decorated with portraits of great Philadelphian physicians (Rush, Shippen, John Redman, J. Morgan, and others, by such famous artists as Charles W. Peale, John Singer Sargent, Benjamin West, and Thomas Eakins).

The building houses one of the country's finest medico-pharmaceutical libraries. It contains over 282,000 volumes, including incunabulae and other rare books, such as the 1761 edition of Morgagni's *De Sedibus et Causis Morborum* and a 1628 edition of Harvey's *De Motu Cordis*, one of three principle surviving copies).

The peaceful herb garden next to the building is maintained by the Women's Committee at the College. Visitors are welcome in this intriguing colonial-type botanical garden, a memorial to Owen J. Roberts (1915–1955).

Antique Apothecary Shop Display
250 East Market Street 17403
(717) 848-1587
Owned and operated by the Historical Society of York County;
Douglas Dolan, executive director.

9 A.M. – 5 P.M.   Monday – Saturday
1 P.M. – 5 P.M.   Sunday
Closed New Year's Day, Good Friday, Easter, Thanksgiving, and
Christmas

Adults, $1.00; students (6–13), 50¢; children (under 6), free;
reduced rates for senior citizens; special group rates

This museum, founded in 1895, houses a fine pharmacy exhibition in the
"Street of Shops" with pharmaceutical equipment, tools, patent medicines, and related artifacts.

PUERTO RICO

San Juan–Rio Piedras Campus

Pharmacy Museum
University of Puerto Rico College of Pharmacy
Rio Piedras 00931
(809) 764-5830
Owned and operated by the University of Puerto Rico College of
Pharmacy; Hector A. Lozada, dean, and Nydia King, historian of
pharmacy.

Weekdays during school hours

Free

A large exhibition hall is fitted with solid mahogany fixtures, exhibit
cases, and dioramas. Elegant European drug jars and shelf ware are displayed together with crude drug containers, apothecary utensils, a large
iron mortar, old microscopes, and archival material. Nearly all the artifacts were used or displayed in pharmacies throughout the island during
earlier decades. Probably the most notable single purchase has been the
collection of J. Federico Legrand (1858–1928) who also was the first
professor of pharmacy at the college. Most of the collection was
gathered as a result of efforts by Dean Emeritus Luis Torres Diaz,
whose personal collections of European drug jars are also on display
and can be seen in his office at the college.

SOUTH CAROLINA

Charleston

Early Drug Store Exhibit
360 Meeting Street 29403
(803) 722-2996
Owned and operated by the Charleston Museum; J. Kenneth Jones,
    curator of history and decorative arts, and Donald G. Herold,
    director.

9 A.M. – 5 P.M.   daily

Adults, $1.50; children, 50¢

There is a drugstore restoration among the period rooms in this oldest
museum in the country (founded 1773) to promote natural history and
to preserve historical and antiquarian objects. The fixtures are from the
Poulnot Drug Store of the late nineteenth century. There are medicine
bottles, drug containers, herb packages, nursing bottles, medicine kits,
show globes, tools of the apothecary, and prescription registers. The
museum also features an herbarium.

SOUTH DAKOTA

Brookings

Pharmacy Artifacts Display
Agricultural Heritage Museum
Old Stock Judging Pavillion 57007
(605) 688-6226
Administered by the Office of Cultural Preservation at Pierre and
    located at the South Dakota State University at Brookings; John
    C. Awald, director.

8 A.M. – 5 P.M.   Monday – Friday
Groups and tours by appointment
Weekend and holiday hours, commencing 1981

Free

The museum, founded in 1967, traces the development of agriculture in
a rural state, but also includes a display of drug jars, patent medicines,
apothecary tools, and locally used medical kits, as well as instruments
from the late nineteenth and twentieth century.

Memphis

Julian Drug Store
Memphis Pink Palace Museum
3050 Central Avenue 38111
(901) 454-5600 / 5603
Owned and operated by the University of Tennessee College of
Pharmacy on loan to the museum for twenty years. The museum
is owned and operated by the Memphis Park Commission.

9 A.M. – 5 P.M.   Tuesday – Thursday
9 A.M. – 10 P.M.   Friday, Saturday
1 P.M. – 5 P.M.   Sunday
Closed Monday

Adults, $1.00; senior citizens, children (grades 1–6), and students
(grades 7–12 and college), 75¢; kindergarten and younger, free.
Group rates available.
9 A.M. – 10 A.M.   Saturday, free hour

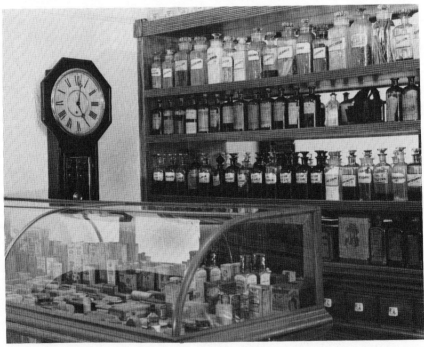

Partial view of a display in the Julian Drug Store which is part of the Memphis
Pink Palace Museum in Tennessee. (Photo courtesy of the Memphis Pink Palace
Museum)

Pharmacist Ralph E. Julian (1886–1975) of Morristown gathered the collection which was transferred to this museum (founded 1928) after his death. It was first opened to the public in 1930 as a museum of natural and cultural history and after recent remodeling, enlargement, and repairs it was reopened in 1977. It displays original fixtures and showcases of the turn of the century, as well as show globes, drug jars, patent medicines, a telephone, and a cash register. It also contains Coca Cola accessories, as well as Orange Crush, Grape Smash, and Hire's Root Beer dispensing apparatus. On display also are tools of the apothecary, a clock, posters, brass light fixtures, herb drawers, and drug percolating and grinding equipment.

TEXAS

Dallas

Doctor's Office and Apothecary Shop
Old City Park—A Museum of Cultural History
1717 Gano Street 75215
(214) 421-5141
Owned and operated by Dallas County Heritage Society, Inc.;
 Louis F. Gorr, director, and Shirley Pettengill, curator of
 collections.

10 A.M. – 4 P.M.   Tuesday – Friday
1:30 P.M. – 4:30 P.M.   Saturday, Sunday (closed Monday)

Adults, $1.00; senior citizens and children, 50¢

A four-room structure including an 1885 doctor's office-residence and waiting room with equipment, furnishings, surgical and examination tables, instruments, obstetric material, medical and saddle bags, and utensils. The adjacent apothecary shop displays drugs, patent medicines, tools, sundries, and shelf ware of the period from 1880–1900. There is also a counseling room with ledgers, journals, and reference and rare books.

Dallas

Health and Drug Exhibits
Dallas Health and Science Museum
Fair Park, First and Forest Avenues
P.O. Box 26407   75226
(214) 428-8351

Owned and operated by the Dallas Health and Science Museum, Inc.; H. Dodson Carmichael, director; Linda Lewis, associate director; and Jack N. McKinney, education coordinator.

9 A.M. – 5 P.M.	Tuesday – Saturday
1 P.M. – 5 P.M.	Sunday and holidays (closed Christmas Day)

Health and Drug Exhibits, free
Planetarium, adults, $1.00; children, 75¢

There are exhibitions on health, alcohol and drug abuse, cell therapy and cancer, reproduction and excretory systems, blood circulation, human physiology and anatomy, general hygiene, and mineralogy.

Dallas

Medico-Pharmaceutical Exhibits
Health Science Center at Dallas
5323 Hines Blvd. 75235
(214) 688-3369
Owned and operated by the University of Texas Health Science Center at Dallas; Dr. Jonathan Erlen, curator.

Weekdays during academic year and by appointment

Free

Several cases have displays of drug jars; microscopes; dental, medical, and surgical instruments; a medical kit; rare medical books; prints; and graphs; as well as some tools of the apothecary.

Houston

Health Exhibition
5800 Caroline Street (second floor)
P.O. Box 88087   77004
(713) 529-3766
Owned and operated by the Foundation for the Museum of Medical Science; Joan Brooks, director.

9:00 A.M. – 4:45 P.M.	Tuesday – Saturday
Noon – 4:45 P.M.	Sunday, Monday

Free; guided tours are provided

There are exhibits on the anatomy and physiology of the human body including a transparent lighted figure, the nervous system, drug abuse, opium pipes, and hypodermic needles.

Jefferson

Medico-Pharmaceutical Exhibit Case
Jefferson Historical Society and Museum
223 West Austin Street, Drawer G   75657
(214) 665-2775
Owned and operated by the Jefferson Historical Society, Inc.; Mrs.
Jack Bullard, curator.

9:30 A.M. – 5:00 P.M.   daily

Adults, $1.00; students, 50¢

The museum is located in an 1888 post office and courthouse building
and was founded in 1948. On display is a showcase with medical instruments and pharmaceutical tools and drug containers.

San Antonio

Medico-Pharmaceutical Exhibition
Durango Boulevard, Hamis Fair Plaza
P.O. Box 1226 78294
(512) 226-7651
Owned and operated by the University of Texas, at San Antonio,
Institute of Texan Cultures; R.H. Shuffler, director, and Laura
Simmons, director of library services.

9 A.M. – 5 P.M.   Tuesday – Friday, September 1 – May 31
1 P.M. – 5 P.M.   Saturday, Sunday, September 1 – May 31
Closed Monday

Free. Guided tours on the hour upon request

Exhibits representing twenty-four ethnic groups and Texan heritage
include a medico-pharmaceutical display. It contains artifacts and illustrations of frontier medical practice and an early Texas apothecary
restoration of fixtures, tools, and pharmaceutical vessels and glassware.

UTAH

Farmington

The Crabtree Drug Store
Utah Pioneer Village
Lagoon Amusement Center 84025
(801) 292-0466
Owned and operated by the National Society Sons of Utah Pioneers. Donated in 1956 by Mr. and Mrs. Horace A. Sorensen,
founders.

| Noon – 10 P.M. | daily, Memorial Day – Labor Day |
| Noon – 10 P.M. | weekends, April 11 – Memorial Day, Labor Day – October 15 |

Free with admission to Amusement Park and $2 purchase of other concessions at Lagoon Amusement Center

This pioneer village of late nineteenth-century Utah known as the "Home of the Praying Oxen" contains thirty-six buildings. One is devoted to a reconstruction of the 1893 drugstore of G.P. Crabtree of 3000 Connor Street, Cairo, Illinois. Beside original fixtures, equipment, and shelf ware, it displays tools of the apothecary, medicine bottles, drug jars, and posters. It was opened May 31, 1961, with Parke, Davis and Company as sponsor, under the auspices of the University of Utah College of Pharmacy 84112, H.H. Wolf, dean.

VERMONT

Shelburne

The Apothecary Shop
Shelburne Museum, U.S. Route 7   05482
(802) 985-3344
Located seven miles south of Burlington. Owned and operated by the Shelburne Museum, Inc.; Benjamin L. Mason, director.

| 9 A.M. – 5 P.M. | daily, May 15 – October 15 |

Adults, $5.00; children (6–16), $2.50
Free parking, cafeteria, and bookshop

This pharmacy reconstruction with authentic fixtures, equipment, and shelf ware contains a large assortment of drug containers, herbs, patent medicines, apothecary tools of the period 1840–1900, posters, and prescriptions. The pharmacy is part of a complex of thirty-five buildings spread over forty-five acres including the offices of a physician and a dentist. Folder on request.

VIRGINIA

Alexandria

Stabler-Leadbeater Apothecary Museum
107 South Fairfax Street 22314
(703) 836-3713
Managed and operated by the Landmark Society of America; Donald C. Slaugh, director.

10 A.M. – 5 P.M.	Monday – Saturday (closed Sunday)
Free	

An authentic collection of antique drugstore furnishings reconstructed in an apothecary shop founded by Edward Stabler in 1792. Son-in-law John Leadbeater joined the Stablers in 1852; the pharmacy remained in the same family until 1933. On display are over 200 hand-blown and British hook-necked bottles with gold-leaf labels, a thermophor (Thermos forerunner), nursing bottles, castor-oil feeders, "perfection" eyeglasses, medicine chests with compartments for leeches, patent medicines, poster, medicinal spoons, labels, ornate drug jars, show globes, and important historical documents. Also shown are pill tiles, show globes, drawers for herbs, and mortars and pestles from the original drugstore building.

Fredericksburg

Hugh Mercer Apothecary Shop
1020 Caroline Street 22401
(703) 373-3362
Located off U.S. 1 and 95 at the corner of Amelia Street. Property of the Association for the Preservation of Virginia Antiquities.

9 A.M. – 5 P.M.	daily, April 1 – October 31
9 A.M. – 4 P.M.	daily, November 1 – March 31

Adults, $1.50; children, 50¢; group rates available

Considered "A Virginia shrine to medicine and pharmacy and to American independence" in which pages of history turn over two centuries in this oldest known original building in America that housed an apothecary shop. It was carefully restored to its original 1764 quaint appearance and architecture and transformed unchanged to a pharmacy museum in 1928.

A native of Aberdeen, Scotland, Dr. Hugh Mercer (ca. 1725–1777) was graduated in medicine from Aberdeen University Marishal College in 1744, and migrated to this country in 1746 to practice the healing art. He served also as a soldier and patriot and entered the Revolutionary Army in 1776 as brigadier general and gave his life on the battlefield a year later at Princeton, New Jersey.

It was common in early America to combine the practice of medicine and pharmacy, and doctors often set up an apothecary shop with a medical office and surgery adjoining the shop as did Dr. Mercer and his partners in Fredericksburg from 1771 until he entered the army five years later.

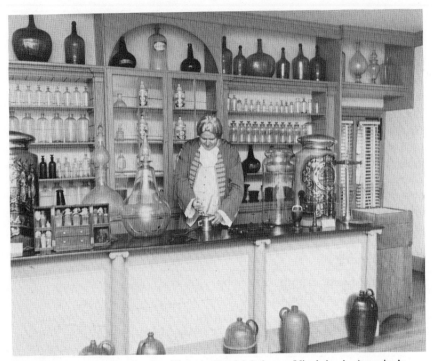

The Hugh Mercer Apothecary Shop in Fredricksburg, Virginia, is America's oldest known drugstore. The building has been restored to its original design with period collections as shown in this view of the interior of the shop.

On display are period pharmacy equipment and tools, the workshop and living quarters. There are faded prescriptions and yellow-leaved ledgers in addition to curious and gleaming gold-labeled bottles and old showcases. Preserved archival materials include accounts written by George Washington, who visited the apothecary shop of his friend Dr. Mercer frequently, using the adjacent sitting room and candle-lit library as an office while in Fredericksburg. A recipe in Mercer's handwriting is also preserved in the shop, as well as John Marshall's cabinet, a blue poison bottle picturing a skull, distilling apparatus, an alcohol lamp used in cupping, and glass-covered species jars.

Williamsburg

Pasteur-Galt Apothecary Shop
Colonial Williamsburg, Duke of Gloucester Street 23185
(804) 229-1000

Located midway between Raleigh Tavern and the colonial Capitol. Administered by the Colonial Williamsburg Foundation for an on-site preservation of the capital of Virginia (founded in 1926); W.A. Hammes, assistant director and supervisor of craft shops.

9 A.M. – 5 P.M.   daily, fall and winter
9 A.M. – 7 P.M.   daily, spring and summer

(Subject to Change):
1-day ticket—adults, $8.50; child, $4.25
2-day ticket—adult, $13.00; child, $6.50
3-day ticket—adult, $16.00; child, $6.50

Virginia's capital flourishes again as a vivid recreation of the American past. Among the eighty-eight preserved and restored historic buildings (dates ranging from 1693–1837) is the apothecary shop reconstructed on the original foundation. It was opened during the observance of "Pharmacy Week" in 1950. The furnishings are of the type that would have been found in a similar eighteenth-century shop. Over the entrance hangs a combination mortar and pestle and staff of Aesculapius sign,

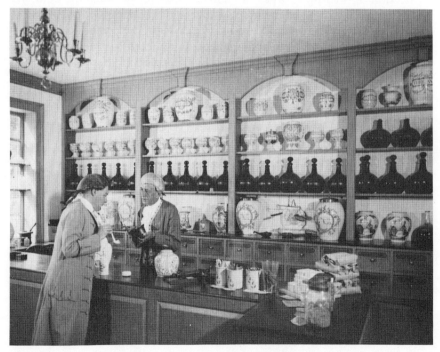

The Pasteur-Galt Apothecary Shop in Colonial Williamsburg where scenes of pharmacy during the period of the American Revolution are reenacted.

representative of the healing arts of pharmacy and medicine. The latter is depicted from a letter's seal found tucked into the wall of the Taylor House on Nicholson Street. The shop is named in memory of two physician-surgeon-pharmacists of Williamsburg.

The first is William J. Pasteur, son of a barber and wigmaker. After the completion of his apprenticeship with Dr. George Gilmer (practiced 1731–1757), he was trained at St. Thomas Hospital in London. He established his practice here when he returned in 1757 and continued until his death in 1791.

The second is John Minson Galt, son of a silversmith, who apprenticed to Pasteur before completing his medical education and training abroad. He was a partner of Dr. Pasteur from 1775–1778 and continued his practice until his death in 1808. Both served as physicians-surgeons during the Revolutionary War.

On display are period furnishings and shelf ware ornamented with rare European drug and leech jars, hand-blown glass bottles, carboys, an old British microscope, pill tiles, herbs in drawers, imported medicines and elixirs, and cardboard pillboxes. Also displayed are Dr. Galt's collection of favorite "cures" of elixirs and drops, personal memorabilia and surgical instruments including a tourniquet, lancets, scarificators, scalpels, forceps, and metallic sounds inserted in the urether for the extraction of kidney and bladder stones, in addition to nineteenth-century surgical instruments in their velvet-lined cases. Other pharmaceutical tools, furnishings, and prints include a late eighteenth-century balance, a marble mortar and pestle sign, and an ointment slab. The back room served as a doctor's office.

WASHINGTON

Olympia

State Pharmaceutical Museum
Washington State Capitol Museum
211 West 21st Avenue 98501
(206) 753-2580
Owned and operated by the Washington State Pharmaceutical
    Association, 1402 Third Avenue, Suite 517, Seattle 98101;
    telephone: (206) 624-4818; R.A. Olson, executive director.

9 A.M. – 5 P.M.   Tuesday – Friday
9 A.M. – noon   Saturday
Special tours on request

Free; donations accepted

Authentic fixtures and equipment of the Casper Heussy Drug Company, located in downtown Seattle since the turn of this century. The equipment was shipped from New York around the Horn to Seattle. It contains drug bottles, pharmacy tools, and other pharmaceutical objects and curios from other pharmacists in the area, which were purchased, collected, and installed by the Washington State Pharmaceutical Association. The museum was opened to the public in 1970 at the Washington State Board of Pharmacy and in 1976 at the Washington State Capitol Museum on loan.

WEST VIRGINIA

Harpers Ferry

Henry Wolff Pharmacy
Department of the Interior, National Park Service
Corner of Shenandoah and High Streets
P.O. Box 65, Harpers Ferry National Historical Park 25425
(304) 535-6371
Hilda E. Staubs, museum technician. On loan from the Smithsonian Institution's National Museum of American History (formerly the National Museum of History and Technology), Washington, D.C. 20560.

8 A.M. – 5 P.M.   daily, winter season
8 A.M. – 8 P.M.   daily, summer season
Closed New Year's Day and Christmas

Free

Among over thirty restored historical buildings and Civil War fortifications is the Henry Wolff (ca. 1818–1891) reconstructed pharmacy. Furnishings and shelving were the authentic fixtures of his original pharmacy built at Union City, New Jersey, in 1884. It continued in service until 1968 when it was donated to the Smithsonian's National Museum of American History by pharmacists Dorothy Specker Pucci, granddaughter of the founder, and her husband (*Pharmacy in History*, 19, 1977, pp. 109-14). Shelf ware, show globes, work apparatus, pharmaceutical artifacts, books, and utensils were assembled by William Stuck, Harry Schrader, and loans from the Smithsonian Institution.

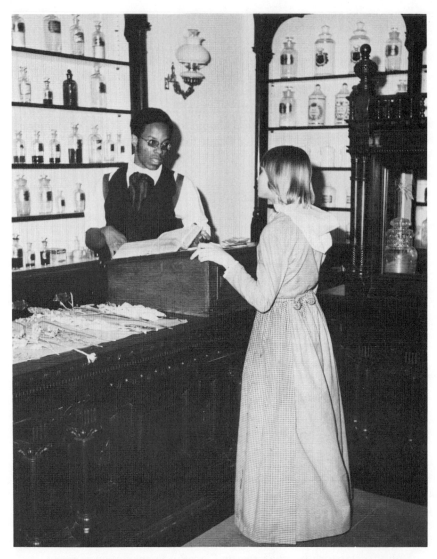

Interior of the Henry Wolff pharmacy at Harpers Ferry National Historical Park in West Virginia, which has the authentic fixtures of Wolff's original pharmacy built at Union City, New Jersey, in 1884. The apprentice and a client in the picture capture the spirit of the period. (Photo courtesy of Harpers Ferry National Historical Park)

Morgantown

Cook-Hayman Pharmacy Museum
Medical Center, Room 1132
West Virginia University School of Pharmacy 26506
(304) 293-5101
Owned and operated by the West Virginia University School of Pharmacy; Art Jacknowitz and John Mayers, curators; Louis A. Luzzi, dean.

8:15 A.M. – 5:00 P.M.   Monday – Friday, and by special appointment

Free

The museum is named after Roy Bird Cook, a prominent West Virginia pharmacist, and Lester Hayman, a former dean of the School of Pharmacy. The elegant 1890 fixtures were made in Baltimore, Maryland, and some of the artifacts came from Charles Town, West Virginia. The medicine chests are gifts from a West Virginia surgeon who served on the SS *Maine.* On display also are patent medicines, glassware, and drug jars, perfume containers, herbs, tools and equipment, and rare pharmaceutical books.

WISCONSIN

Cassville

Rydell Apothecary Shop
Stonefield, Box 486, at the Nelson Dewey State Park Complex 53806
(608) 725-5210
Located on the Mississippi river, about 35 miles south of Prairie du Chien on Wisconsin 81 and 133. Owned and operated by the Wisconsin State Historical Society, 816 State Street, Madison 53706; Melvin L. Houghton, historic-site manager.

9 A.M. – 5 P.M.   daily, May – October
Tickets sold 9 A.M. – 4:30 P.M.; group tours by arrangement.

Adults, $3.50; students (5–17) $1.00. Group rates by advance reservation, 20 percent discount; students and educational groups, $1.00 each.

This shop is part of a re-creation of a late nineteenth-century Wisconsin village. It is a free-standing drugstore restoration of the late nineteenth and early twentieth centuries. Fixtures were moved from the Rydell

Drug Store at Superior, Wisconsin. Most of the artifacts, however, came from the Rydell and Fred Mink store in Cassville. Shelves are stocked with ingredients for the making of sundry medicines, salves and ointments, drug bottles and jars, as well as tools and equipment of the apothecary. Plans call for the opening of a new building that will house manufacturing machines and equipment acquired from the defunct Willson–Monarch laboratories of pharmaceutical and culinary products. The exhibition also includes a cigar maker, confectionary and ice cream equipment, an 1890 operational pill-making machine for "cure all" medications, drug grinders, and mixers.

Among other related exhibits beside agriculture and dairy products is a doctor's office copied from one occupied by a Dr. Martin of Kewaunee about 1880 with furnishings and medical instruments and equipment from Dr. Alfred Belitz of Pepin, Wisconsin.

Milwaukee

Laab's Apothecary Exhibition (The Apotheke)
Milwaukee Public Museum
800 West Wells Street 53233
(414) 278-2700

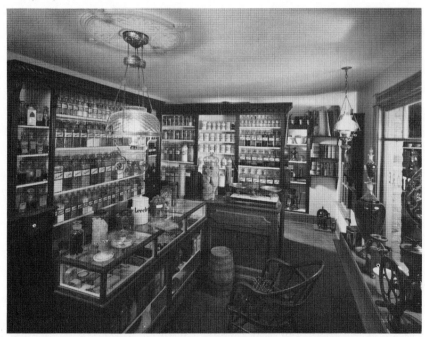

Laab's apothecary shop is a replica of a Milwaukee, Wisconsin, store around the turn of the century which contains original period fixtures and shelf ware. (Photo courtesy of the Milwaukee Public Museum.)

Owned and operated by Milwaukee County; Donald Hoke, assistant curator, History Department.

9 A.M. – 5 P.M.   daily
Closed certain holidays

Milwaukee County residents, adults, $1.00; children, 25¢ (free on Monday)
Others: adults, $2.00; children 75¢.
Group rate for out-of-county groups with a minimum of 20 persons

This charming drugstore replica along the museum's "Streets of Old Milwaukee" represents the period 1890–1910. On display are show globes, leech and gold-labeled drug jars, cobalt-blue bottles, patent medicines, shelf ware and tools of the apothecary from several donations including the Otto Laab pharmacy fixtures and artifacts.

Nearby is another exhibit of a period oculist's shop with tools and equipment, spectacles and furnishings, illustrating some aspects of the history of American ophthalmology.

Milwaukee

Yesterday's Drugstore
Milwaukee County Historical Center
910 North Third Street 53203
(414) 273-8288
Owned and operated by the Milwaukee County Historical Society; Miss Kathleen O'Hara, publications and public contact, and Harry H. Anderson, executive director.

9 A.M. – 5 P.M.   Monday – Saturday
1 P.M. – 5 P.M.   Sunday
Closed on major national holidays

Free

"Yesterday's Drugstore" represents pharmacy at the turn of the century. It features tools of the trade, counter scales, drug mills, apothecary jars, tinctures, cork and pill presses, mortars and pestles, a Diamond Dye cabinet, posters, mirrored prescription counter, show globes, a cash register, and patent medicines. The entire display was donated by the family of Theodore Marlewski, a Milwaukee druggist, after his death. The attractive custom-built fixtures were made in Milwaukee by a Polish cabinetmaker in the 1880s.

In addition, there is a doctor's office of about 1900 which represents Dr. Nicholas Senn's (1844–1908) clinic. On display are an examining table, laboratory equipment, surgical instruments, sterilizing unit, diplomas and books, as well as medical kits, utensils, and remedies. A case exhibit sponsored by the County Medical Association and opened to the public in 1977 features county doctors including women (represented by a photograph of Laura Ross Walcott, 1834–1915, first woman physician to practice in Wisconsin) and black physicians (represented by Allen L. Herron who practiced medicine for fifty years).

The medico-pharmaceutical exhibits are equipped with a series of push-button panels that illuminate to give the viewer information about important artifacts and pharmaceutical utensils and furnishings and how they were used at the time. There is also a panel to compare and contrast today's pharmacy with that of yesteryear, with the viewer's attention drawn to a symbolic sign that reads "pure drugs and chemicals—prescriptions carefully compounded."

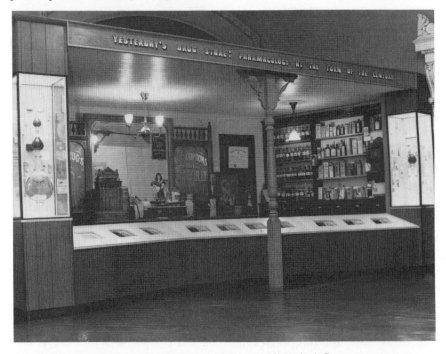

Yesterday's Drugstore at the Milwaukee County Historical Center portrays a pharmacy of 1900. Nearly every item in the re-created shop was collected by Theodore Marlewski, a Milwaukee, Wisconsin, pharmacist. (Photo courtesy of the Milwaukee County Historical Society)

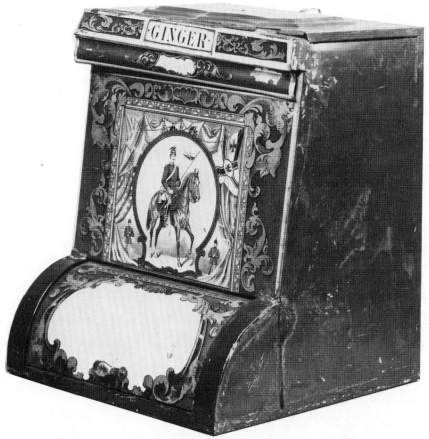

An American tin spice dispenser used in a nineteenth-century Midwest pharmacy to dispense ginger. (Photo courtesy of Kremers Reference Files, School of Pharmacy, University of Wisconsin)

Pharmacy Museums and Exhibitions in Canada

The following entries are arranged alphabetically according to provinces and then subdivided according to cities and towns within each province.

ALBERTA

Calgary

Gledhill's Drug Store
Heritage Park, 1900 Heritage Drive S.W. T2V 2X3
Owned by the City of Calgary and operated by the Heritage Park
Society; W.J. Campbell, manager.

10 A.M. – 6 P.M.   daily, Victoria Day (mid-May) holiday weekend until Labor Day; weekends only from Labor Day until the Canadian Thanksgiving Day holiday on the second Monday in October.

Adults, $2; children (3–14), $1

Heritage Park aims to depict life on the Canadian prairies before and after the development of the national railway in 1885 and before World War I in 1914. The drugstore in the park is one built originally in 1908 by F.E. Livingstone at Dundurn and subsequently relocated in Hanley, Saskatchewan. The interior boasts solid-oak fixtures ornamented with semi-Corinthian engraved pillars, a solid maple floor, and a ceiling of embossed tin. The pharmaceutical artifacts were collected for the project by the Alberta Pharmaceutical Association, Glenbow Museum, and Heritage Park.

Edmonton

Daly's Drug Store
Fort Edmonton Park
Located in the pre-railway settlement area at the west end of Quesnell Bridge.

Owned by the City of Edmonton, Parks and Recreation
Department; Dr. Howard Welch, senior historical researcher.

10 A.M. – 6 P.M.   daily, Victoria Day – Labor Day
1 P.M. – 5 P.M.   weekends, Labor Day – early October
School and special tours by arrangement

Adults, $2.75, students (13–17); senior citizens (65 and over), $1.50;
children (6–12), $1.00; family group (two adults and their children under 18), $7.00.
Group rates, same charges as above, except pre-booked groups of
10–29 receive 20 percent discount; prebooked groups of 30 and
over receive 25 percent discount.

Daly's Drug Store re-creates a pharmacy on a street typical of 1885, one
of six major areas in the ambitious Ford Edmonton Park development
which plans eventually to re-create settlements of various time periods
from about 1845 to the present. Another pharmacy is planned for a 1905
street. The Daly Drug Store combines the store with a dispensary,
doctor's office, and doctor's residence. The practice was established
originally in 1882 by Dr. H.C. Wilson, who had come from Ontario. He
continued to practice medicine at the back of the premises until the
1890s, although he had sold the pharmacy in 1885 to Philip Daly of Fort
Rouge, Manitoba. The professional practice aspects of the pharmacy
have been re-created to represent the eclectic conditions that often
prevailed in early pharmacies on the western frontier, prior to the completion of a national railway.

BRITISH COLUMBIA

Barkerville

J.P. Taylor Drug Store
Barkerville Historic Park V0K 1B0
(604) 994-3209
Owned and operated by the government of British Columbia,
Ministry of Lands, Parks, and Housing.

8:00 A.M. – dusk   daily

Free

Barkerville Historic Park re-creates the gold-rush town of Barkerville,
British Columbia, as it was about 1869–1885. The J.P. Taylor Drug
Store which operated at this time has been reconstructed with particular
help from the South Vancouver Island Pharmacists' Association and the

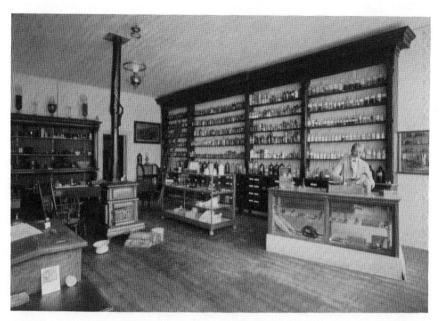

Interior of the J.P. Taylor Drug Store in Barkerville Historic Park which is a re-creation of the gold-rush town of Barkerville of over a century ago. (Photo by Dorse McTaggart)

British Columbia Pharmaceutical Association. Most of the shelf ware and fixtures came from the Thomas Shotbolt pharmacy in Victoria, British Columbia, one of the earliest pharmacies in the area that closed after a century of operation. One of the nostalgic ties with the Barkerville pharmacy's past is a stagecoach schedule found in a copy of the 1862 *U.S. Dispensatory* known to have come originally from the J.P. Taylor shop.

Burnaby

Finlayson's Pharmacy *and*
Way San Yuen Wat Kee and Company (Chinese herbalist's shop)
Heritage Village, Century Park Museum Association
4900 Deer Lake Avenue V5G 3T6
(604) 291-8525
Located off Canada Way at Gilpin (leave TransCanada 401 at
    Sperling South Exit). Operated by the Century Park Museum
    Association, a nonprofit registered society, on behalf of the
    Corporation of the District of Burnaby; John Adams, curator.

10 A.M. – 6 P.M.	daily, summer
10 A.M. – 6 P.M.	Saturday, Sunday, spring and fall
Afternoons only, winter; open all year for school and other tours	

Adults, $1; children (under 12) and senior citizens, 50¢; children (under 6), free

Finlayson's Pharmacy has a general collection of pharmacy artifacts from the period 1890–1920, housed in a reconstructed building. The collection, gathered from pharmacies throughout British Columbia's Lower Mainland region, features apothecary globes, a set of rosewood herbal drawers, and Delft apothecary jars, as well as a wide range of glass storage bottles. A small archive is maintained containing prescription books and letter books from area pharmacies. The display was established with assistance from the University of British Columbia School of Pharmacy and the Lower Mainland Pharmacists Association.

Way San Yuen Wat Kee and Company (Chinese herbalist's shop): The display consists of the entire contents of a Chinese herbalist's shop reassembled in a reconstructed structure. The original business opened in Victoria, British Columbia, about 1903 and continued until 1970. The display represents a traditional herbalist's of the Canton region as it would have been from at least the mid-nineteenth century. It features a set of mahogany and rosewood herbal drawers with hand carving, a complete range of hand-manufacturing equipment, and herb containers, all from China.

Fort Steele

Pioneer Drug Hall
Fort Steele Historic Park V0B 1N0
(604) 489-3351
Owned and operated by the Parks Branch of the Ministry of Lands, Parks, and Housing of the Province of British Columbia; Kenneth N. Zurosky, curator.

9 A.M. – 8 P.M.	daily, July and August
9 A.M. – 5 P.M.	May, June, September, October

Free

The pharmacy is a reconstruction of the "Pioneer Drug Hall" first opened in Fort Steele in 1896 by Arthur W. Bleasdell, who had come originally from Ontario. Artifacts and fixtures are also drawn from another early pharmacy located in Kimberley, British Columbia. The pharmacy is divided into a front shop and a dispensary at the rear.

L.G. Cook Pharmacy
British Columbia Provincial Museum
601 Belleville Street V8W 1A1
(604) 387-3701
M.J. Wright, Modern History Division.

10:00 A.M. – 7:30 P.M.	daily, April 1 – September 30
10:00 A.M. – 5:30 P.M.	daily, October 1 – March 31

Free

The L.G. Cook Pharmacy re-creates a shop of about 1900 and is situated with other similar establishments on a turn-of-the-century street in the museum's Modern History Gallery. Most of the pharmaceutical artifacts on display were donated by the British Columbia Pharmaceutical Association and installed by Bedford Bates, a local practicing pharmacist.

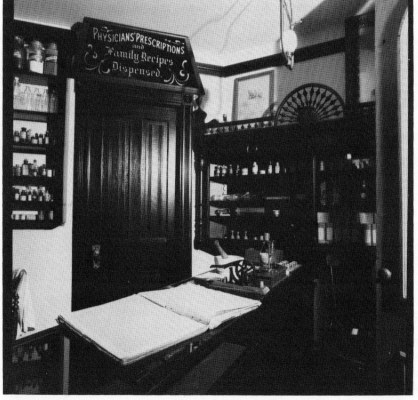

Pharmacy interior of about 1900 in a gallery of the British Columbia Provincial Museum in Victoria.

Winnipeg

1920 Drug Store
Manitoba Museum of Man and Nature, Urban Gallery
190 Rupert Avenue R3B 0N2
(204) 956-2830
Funded by the government of Manitoba, the government of
Canada, and corporate and individual support.

Mid-May – mid-September
10 A.M. – 9 P.M.   Monday – Saturday (including holidays)
Noon – 9 P.M.   Sunday
Mid-September – mid-May
10 A.M. – 5 P.M.   Monday – Friday
10 A.M. – 9 P.M.   Saturday
Noon – 6 P.M.   Sunday, holidays

General, 75¢; family, $3.00 maximum; senior citizens and children
(under six), free.

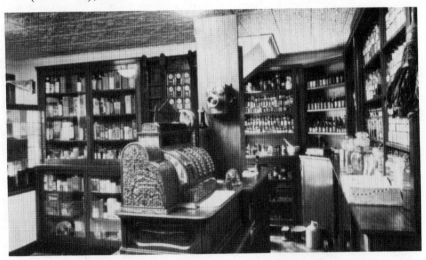

This reconstruction of a drugstore of the 1920s is in the Manitoba Museum of
Man and Nature in Winnipeg, Manitoba. (Photo courtesy of Henry Kalen, Ltd.)

Under the shop sign of "Bletcher & McDougall Drugs," this reconstruction represents pharmacy in a street of the 1920s. In addition to the customary front shop and dispensary stocked with such items as period drugs, proprietaries, and sundries, there is a small post office, and an area for the manufacture of pharmaceutical preparations. Cameras and photographic equipment are, as one would expect, prominent among the artifacts on display. A typical embossed metal ceiling completes the picture. A variety of items are sold in the shop, including postcards, licorice ropes, stick candy, and soaps. The project was carried out with the consultation and active participation of pharmacist C.G. Chapman and a committee of the Manitoba Pharmaceutical Association.

NEWFOUNDLAND

St. John's

Pharmacy Museum
Newfoundland Pharmaceutical Association
205 LeMarchant Road A1C 2H5
(709) 579-3371
J.J. O'Mara, coordinator.

9:00 A.M. – 12:30 P.M. and 1:30 P.M. – 5:00 P.M.   Monday – Friday

Free

The museum contains approximately 1,500 items relating to the history of the association and of pharmacy in Newfoundland. Included are books, artifacts, records, and proprietary remedies. In storage is a complete set of pharmacy fixtures about 100 years old that are planned for the re-creation of a late nineteenth-century pharmacy.

NOVA SCOTIA

Granville Ferry

Louis Hébert Quarters
The Habitation, Port Royal National Historic Park
Annapolis County
(902) 532-5197
Owned and operated by Parks Canada, the Department of Indian and Northern Affairs, the government of Canada; G.R. Bowen, area interpretive officer.

10 A.M. – 5 P.M.	daily, April 1 to June 15
9 A.M. – 8 P.M.	daily, June 15 to Labor Day
10 A.M. – 5 P.M.	daily, Labor Day–October 31

Free

The Habitation at Port Royal, founded in 1605, was the first permanent settlement in North America north of the Spanish settlement of Saint Augustine, Florida. Among those in the pioneering adventure was Louis Hébert, a Parisian apothecary, who thus became the first permanent pharmacist in the New World and is also credited with being the first farmer in Canada when he later settled at what is now Quebec City. The Habitation was reconstructed by the Canadian government in 1938–39. In the room which Hébert apparently shared with the resident surgeon is a drug chest and drug jars and dried herbs of the period, along with some other equipment.

Sherbrooke

Sherbrooke Drug Store
Sherbrooke Village
P.O. Box 285   B0J 3C0
(902) 522-2400
Operated by the Sherbrooke Restoration Commission under the
    direction of the Nova Scotia Museum, Cultural Services Program,
    Department of Education; J.G. Duff, Professor of Pharmacy,
    Dalhousie University, Halifax, Nova Scotia.

| 9:30 A.M. – 5:30 P.M. | daily, May 15 to October 15 |

$1.50

The pharmacy is one of the restored buildings located in the historic Sherbrooke Village. The town was built on the site of a fur-trading post established in 1655, and prospered for many years as a lumbering and ship-building outlet. When gold was discovered in 1861, it enhanced the area's prominence. In this re-creation of a late nineteenth- to early twentieth-century pharmacy, period drugs, proprietary medicines, containers, and equipment are displayed. Most of the artifacts were collected by the College of Pharmacy, Dalhousie University, while some of the fixtures came originally from Ontario. Professor J.G. Duff of the College of Pharmacy was the principal consultant for the project.

ONTARIO

Midland

Apothecary Shop
Sainte-Marie among the Hurons, Huronia Historical Parks,
P.O. Box 160 L4R 4K8
(705) 526-7838
Owned and operated by the Ministry of Culture and Recreation,
the government of the Province of Ontario; Bill Byrick, manager.

10 A.M. – 6 P.M.   daily, Victoria Day – Labor Day (last visitor
admitted 5:15 P.M.)
10 A.M. – 5 P.M.   daily, Labor Day to Canadian Thanksgiving
(second Monday in October) (last visitor admitted 4:15 P.M.)

Adults, $1.50; students, 75¢; children, 25¢; adult group rate, $1.25;
family, $3.50.
Prices subject to change

Sainte-Marie was built in 1639 as the central residence of the Jesuit
Mission to the Huron Indians. It was the only European settlement in
Canada east of Quebec and Three Rivers, 800 miles away. Sainte Marie
was abandoned and destroyed by the missionaries in 1649 when adversi-
ties became insurmountable. It has now been reconstructed and a new
interpretative museum serves as its main entrance. A small (10 ×
16-foot) extension of the hospital has been restored as the pharmacy and
is stocked with purgatives and other herbs used for the treatment of
colds and sore throats; some tools of the apothecary are also displayed
in the interpretative museum. The shop is reputed to be the earliest
pharmacy established in inland Canada and the northern United States.
The apothecary, Joseph Molère, who was on duty in Sainte-Marie during the period of its existence, 1639–1649, also assisted the settlement's
surgeon.

Minesing

1890 Pharmacy
Simocoe County Museum
R.R. #2 L0L 1Y0
(705) 728-3721
Minesing is located 5 miles north of Barrie, Ontario, on Highway
26.
Owned and operated by the County of Simcoe; B. Cameron,
director.

9 A.M. – 5 P.M.	daily, Monday – Saturday
1 P.M. – 5 P.M.	Sunday
1 P.M. – 6:30 P.M.	weekends, July and August

Adults, $1; senior citizens, 75¢; students, 50¢; children, 25¢

The pharmacy re-creation is part of a village street of 1890 in the main building of the museum. Artifacts on display date from about 1870 to the turn of the century and have been collected from the area around Barrie.

Niagara-on-the-Lake

Niagara Apothecary
Corner King and Queen Streets
P.O. Box 903   L0S 1J0
(416) 468-3845, seasonal only; (416) 962-4861, off season
Owned by the Ontario Heritage Foundation, Ministry of Culture
    and Recreation, the government of the Province of Ontario;
    operated by the Ontario College of Pharmacists (provincial
    licensing body); Ernst W. Stieb, curator.

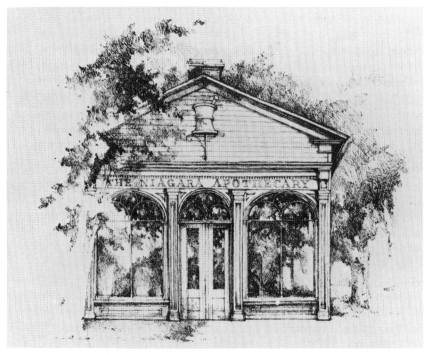

The Niagara Apothecary has been authentically restored on a site where a pharmacy was first opened in 1866. (Drawing by Robert Montgomery of Exterior)

Noon – 6 P.M.   daily, mid-May — Labor Day

Free

Authentic restoration, by Canada's foremost restoration architect, Peter Stokes, of a pharmacy that first opened on these premises in 1866, after having been at other locations in the town since the early nineteenth century. It is the only building surviving from this period in this historically and architecturally notable area. Fixtures are of black walnut and butternut and there are replicas of the original crystal chandeliers. Much of the original glass and ceramic ware, reputedly imported from England about 1830, survives. Other artifacts date from about that period to about 1900. Original prescription and account records are from about 1830. Rotating exhibits from other collections are incorporated into the permanent collection of artifacts during each season. The mid-Victorian exterior is dominated by gracefully arched Florentine windows and a large gilt mortar-and-pestle shop sign.

Toronto

History of Medicine Museum
Academy of Medicine, Toronto
288 Bloor Street West M5S 1V8
(416) 922-1134
Located at the corner of Huron Street, entrance off Huron. Owned and operated by the Academy of Medicine, Toronto; John Senior, curator.

Weekdays by appointment

Free

In spacious refurbished quarters in a turn-of-the-century mansion, the museum presently consists of three main sections. One area is devoted to paleopathology, the center of attention being the Toronto autopsy of 1974 of Nakht, a 3,200-year-old Egyptian mummy. The second area focuses upon the history of Canadian medicine and includes the natural history cabinet of the Reverend W.A. Johnson, one of Sir William Osler's early mentors. The third main area is given over to the artifacts of the remarkable T.G.H. Drake Collection. Although primarily a pediatric collection, the Drake Collection boasts a fine assortment of English delft pill tiles and drug jars, as well as mortars and pestles, coins and tokens, medicine chests, medicine spoons, pill boxes, pewter enema syringes, and medicinal caricatures. A printed catalog is presently in preparation.

QUEBEC

Quebec City

Musée de l'Hôtel-Dieu de Québec
(Museum of the Hôtel-Dieu Hospital)
rue des Remparts
(418) 692-2492, extension 47
Owned and operated by the Soeurs Hospitalières de St. Augustin;
Sister Morin, curator.

9 A.M. – 11 A.M.   daily except Sunday morning
2 P.M. – 5 P.M.   daily
To enter, ring bell at entrance gate

Free; appointments requested for groups of ten or more persons.

The museum consists of a truly remarkable, if somewhat disparate, collection of such things as medical and pharmaceutical equipment and containers, photographs, manuscripts, etc., dating back to 1639, when the hospital was first established. It is the oldest hospital in North America and one of the oldest in the British Commonwealth. When circumstances permit, visitors are also shown some of the oldest extant sections of the building. *NOTE: A passable working knowledge of French is desirable to appreciate exhibit captions and to communicate with museum attendants.*

SASKATCHEWAN

North Battleford

Drug Store
Western Development Museum and Pioneer Village
Box 183, North Battleford, Saskatchewan S9A 2Y1
(306) 445-8033
Located at junction of highways 16 and 40 east

8 A.M. – 6 P.M.   daily, May
8 A.M. – 8 P.M.   daily, June, September
8 A.M. – 9 P.M.   daily, July, August
The main building is open 9 A.M. – 5 P.M. Monday – Friday,
    October 1 – April 30, but the Pioneer Village is closed.

Adults, $1.50; children, 50¢; family, $4.00
Western Development Museum's season family pass to all four
    branches, $5

The pharmacy is one of about thirty buildings in the Pioneer Village. The setting re-creates a shop of the early 1900s and is well stocked with items of that era.

Saskatoon

Coad's Drug Store
Saskatoon Branch, Saskatchewan Western Development Museums
P.O. Box 1910, 2610 Lorne Avenue South S7K 3S5
(306) 652-8900
Robert Bruce Shepard, manager

9 A.M. – 9 P.M.	daily, mid-May – mid-September
9 A.M. – 5 P.M.	weekdays, mid-September – mid-May
Noon – 5 P.M.	weekends and holidays, mid-September – mid-May

Adults, $1.50; Pioneer (over 65), $1.00; children (under 16), 50¢; family, $4.00

Coad's Drug Store is located in the Boomtown Street exhibit of the Saskatoon Branch. It is reminiscent of early prairie pharmacies in western Canada. The collection on display includes a range of early goods, supplies, and business records.

American Pharmacy's Historical Markers

A need to recognize noteworthy sites relating to important events in pharmaceutical history in the United States has been felt for over two decades. Historical markers placed at such sites would serve as reminders of some of the contributions that the profession, the pharmaceutical industry, and pharmacy's educational institutions have made to public health and welfare. Toward achieving this end, a committee on historical markers was formed during the 1958 annual meeting of the American Institute of the History of Pharmacy.

In 1959, the Institute's Council adopted a recommendation by this committee to implement a project "to mark and permanently recognize historical sites meaningful to American Pharmacy." Procedural outlines for implementing the program were prepared, and pharmacists and pharmaceutical groups and organizations were encouraged to recommend specific sites for historical markers—to be reviewed by a committee and approved by the Council.[1] The first such site was marked three years later, in 1963.

The following is an annotated list of markers dedicated by the American Institute of the History of Pharmacy at historical sites from 1963 through 1980.

1. October 10, 1963: Site of the pharmacy of Louis Joseph Dufilho, at 514 Chartres Street, New Orleans, Louisiana—in the heart of the old French Quarter—and known as *La Pharmacie Française*. Pharmacist Dufilho is recognized as one of the first pharmacists to be licensed in the United States. The plaque mounted just to the right of the doorway gives permanent recognition to pharmacy's vital significance for the improvement of public health. It symbolizes the beginning (1816) of a system of certifying professional competence of pharmacists in the United States, establishing an important principle by which the profession would eventually be recognized and regulated.[2] On this historical site, a pharmacy museum, one of the finest showcases of its kind in the country, was reconstituted and is open to the public (for description see page 47).

2. October 2, 1964: Site of founding of the American Pharmaceutical Association in Philadelphia, Pennsylvania, on October 7, 1852. The plaque was placed on a stone column to the left of the main entrance of the Lit Brothers Department Store, located at 8th (near Filbert, then 710 Zane) and Market streets in the heart of downtown Philadelphia. Here was the original building of the Philadelphia College of Pharmacy where the American Pharmaceutical Association, the first and principal national professional society of pharmacists in this country, was founded.[3] The building was demolished in 1980, and plans for the replacement of the marker are currently uncertain.

3. January 22, 1966: Site of founding of the American Institute of the History of Pharmacy on January 22, 1941. This event occurred in the old chemistry-pharmacy building (now Chamberlin Hall) at the University of Wisconsin at Madison (corner of University Avenue and Charter Street). It is stated on the plaque that the institute was founded to help cultivate pharmacy's role in the history of human civilization, and to promote the humanistic and aesthetic values of the profession.[4]

4. October 18, 1967: Founding site of the University of Michigan Department of Pharmacy, which was consequential as the first in a state university. The plaque, installed at the College of Pharmacy Building at Ann Arbor, Michigan, commemorates physician-chemist Albert B. Prescott's introduction of the state university's pharmaceutical curriculum which was authorized in 1868. The Department of Pharmacy became a School of Pharmacy in 1876. The pharmacy curriculum at Michigan pioneered bold new concepts that eventually transformed American pharmaceutical education. Michigan introduced extensive laboratory instruction coupled with basic science, making the academic study of pharmacy practically a full-time occupation.[5]

5. May 19, 1972: Founding site of the Rho Chi Society, the national honor society of pharmacy which was chartered 1922. The plaque was installed at the old chemistry-pharmacy building at the University of Michigan at Ann Arbor on the fiftieth anniversary of the society and recognizes its contribution to the encouragement of scientific research and high educational standards in pharmacy in the United States.[6]

6. August 2, 1974: Founding site of the University of Wisconsin's School of Pharmacy at Madison in 1883. The plaque was placed on South Hall, the original home of the Department of Pharmacy. The marker recognizes the school's national influence and its pioneering role in establishing the first four-year baccalaureate as a professional degree in pharmacy—first awarded in 1895—and the first Ph.D. as a research degree in pharmaceutical specialities in the United States which was first awarded in 1902. Both programs were pioneered by pharmacist-educator Edward Kremers.[7]

7. January 24, 1976: Site of the establishment in 1778 of a manufacturing pharmacy and "issuing store" for the Revolutionary forces by Apothecary-General Andrew Craigie. The marker was placed on a stone boulder on the grounds of the Army War College, Carlisle, Pennsylvania.[8]

8. June 12, 1976: Founding site of the pharmacy of the Pennsylvania Hospital at Philadelphia, established in 1752 as the first hospital pharmacy in the thirteen colonies. The plaque was placed on the doorway of the room in the historic Pine Building that served as a part of the pharmacy at its second location, from 1800–1927, which is presently the office of the hospital's president. The first appointed apothecary was Jonathan Roberts, followed in 1755 by John Morgan. Here medications were prepared daily as prescribed by the attending physicians, illustrating the need for professional pharmaceutical skills and services in providing adequate treatment and cures for the sick.[9]

9. July 10, 1976: Site of the compilation of the "Lititz Pharmacopoeia." The marker was placed at the entrance of the Brothers' House of the Moravian Church, built in 1759, which was used from December 1777 to August 1778 as a hospital for the Continental troops during the Revolutionary War. The "Lititz Pharmacopoeia," for the use of the medical department of the army, was prepared by Physician-General William Brown at Lititz and published in Philadelphia in 1778. It was the first American formulary—a pioneer effort at the standardization of drug formulas in this country.[10]

10. September 5, 1980: Site of the Northern Regional Research Laboratory, United States Department of Agriculture, where key contributions were made to the development of large-scale penicillin production in the 1940s. These included the introduction of submerged culture fermentation, the use of precursors to produce more effective penicillin, and the discovery of a mold strain more productive of penicillin.

Notes

1. *Pharmacy in History,* vol. 4 (1959), pp. 58 and 72 and vol. 5 (1960), pp. 59-60.
2. Ibid., vol. 8 (1966), pp. 79-81; or "Réflexions sur une vieille pharmacie américaine," *Revue d'Histoire de la pharmacie,* vol. 52 (1964), 107-108.
3. *Pharmacy in History,* vol. 9 (1967), pp. 14, 22-24.
4. Ibid., pp. 45, 51.
5. Ibid., vol. 10 (1968), pp. 14-15.
6. Ibid., vol. 14 (1972), 116-117.
7. Ibid., vol. 16 (1974), 159-160.
8. Ibid., vol. 18 (1976), pp. 69-71.
9. Ibid., vol. 19 (1977), pp. 50-53.
10. Ibid.

Concluding Remarks

In the fall of 1913, the State Historical Society of Wisconsin installed in its museum in Madison a reconstructed unit of a "historical drug store" representing pharmacy in Wisconsin from 1848–1898: "The first half century of statehood." This was apparently the first educational pharmacy museum in North America devoted entirely to a drugstore restoration open to the public. It resulted from the untiring effort of pharmacist-author-educator Edward Kremers (1865–1941), whose influence on the development of historical pharmacy in the New World can hardly be exaggerated.[1] Since then, a sense of intellectual curiosity and appreciation has swept the pharmaceutical scene throughout the continent. Professionals, educators, and the public have become more aware and appreciative than ever before of their heritage and the aesthetic value of pharmaceutical antiques.

As a result of this new awareness, there are now more than 138 medico-pharmaceutical museums or exhibitions in the United States and 18 in Canada that are on special or semipermanent display open to the public. To those can be added many others, including noteworthy collections of private collectors, antique dealers, art galleries, and offices of professionals, educators, and manufacturers of medico-pharmaceutical products.[2] Also, some collections privately owned or stored in research and study quarters in large museums contain rare and significant pharmaceutical objects and equipment and compare favorably with the already described museum restorations and pharmaceutical displays open to the public. There are, in addition, several strictly medical or health museums devoted to education concerning contemporary health problems and for the teaching of such things as human anatomy and physiology that were excluded from the present survey.

This survey of North American pharmacy museums raises a number of questions, such as: How are these "temples of the muses" on our pharmaceutical heritage distributed geographically? What is their mission? What impact do they have on the profession and the public at large?

Among the 50 states of the union, 43 have one or more such historical exhibitions, plus two in the District of Columbia and one in Puerto Rico. There has been a tremendous total increase of 48 museums over the 1972 survey. In Canada there are 18 museums distributed in cities within eight provinces. Serious efforts are being reported to increase the number of such restorations in states and provinces in order to preserve pharmacy's past, especially in those areas that have no public exhibits yet. Ranking high among the states and provinces having the greatest number of museums are: New York State with 15 museums, Massachusetts, 9; California, Pennsylvania, and Ohio, 7 each; Texas, Georgia, and Michigan, 6 each; and Connecticut and British Columbia (Canada), 5 each.

It is hoped that through the publication of this guidebook many educators, administrators, and leaders in pharmacy will show more concern and increase their cooperation in this endeavor. It seems imperative to give some priority to preserving the remarkable heritage to which we are all indebted. Expert consultation and direction concerning collecting, restoring, and exhibiting is available through the American Institute of the History of Pharmacy and the Smithsonian Institution, as well as from individual historians and friends of the profession's past. It is further hoped that each state and province in North America will have an active part to play in reviving, honoring, and perpetuating a worthy heritage.[3]

The aims of these museums are self-evident: to create interest in and genuine appreciation of pharmacy's past, to trace esthetic and techno-scientific development in the art of the apothecary as a member of the health professions, and to educate the public in the "mystery and art of the apothecary."

Sponsorship and Resources

A significant number of the public exhibitions surveyed constitute a part of larger museums and galleries, while others are managed by historical societies of the medical profession which consider pharmacy a part of the healing arts. What about pharmacy schools and state societies? Most colleges had at one time or another or would like to have historical exhibits on their premises. State societies, likewise, often would like to help. Four problems, however, arise in this connection that prevent the fulfillment of such high hopes.

1. Lack of space: Colleges are in dire need of office and laboratory space; thus it is difficult to set aside space for a historical exhibit. In some cases, already existing pharmaco-historical exhibits may have been dismantled because of space needs.

2. Lack of personnel: As often is the case, it is difficult to find in the colleges a qualified faculty member who has the interest, time, and opportunity to make a historical display vibrant, alive, and intriguing to attract the attention and respect of colleagues, students, and the public

at large. State pharmaceutical societies, being involved in contemporary professional problems, generally do not have the time or personnel to pay attention to matters of this nature.

3. Lack of finances: To build and maintain a pharmacy museum involves considerable financial expenses. Most colleges weigh this goal against other research and educational projects and give the latter priority.

4. Lack of appreciation of the value of history: To many the scientific and business sides of the profession outweigh that of the cultural, aesthetic, and humanistic, so that interest in supporting a museum diminishes.

Now what of the pharmaceutical industry? Here space, personnel, and finances should not be a problem, especially when compared with the huge sums of money spent on such activities as advertising. Industry is an important and legitimate source of assistance. Most of the large and leading manufacturing companies have roots in nineteenth-century American pharmacy. Therefore, they can repay their debt in honoring that commendable heritage, nourishing its records, and supporting efforts to display its historical artifacts and furnishings. Many have accepted some responsibility, but more involvement is needed, since this concerns not only the profession's past, but the aims and aspirations for a brighter future. History revives a sense of cultural pride in one's professional heritage.[4]

Avenues to Progress

Pharmacy and health museums in Northern America have developed and progressed in many respects, but there is still much to be done. It is the author's conclusion that some active steps should be taken to secure and improve the quality, maintenance, and increase of these "emissaries" of good will on behalf of pharmacy and its cultural history. The following recommendations are offered.

1. Relating to the profession: One cannot stress enough the importance of pharmacy's humanistic role as a profession dedicated to safeguarding national health. The highly qualified and dedicated pharmacist, whether researcher, writer, practitioner, or educator can make a significant contribution to the preservation of the heritage of his profession. As a member of the public at large, he can support and actively participate in organized societies such as the American Institute of the History of Pharmacy which are dedicated to preserving a great legacy. There should be no place for indifference in appreciating the pharmaceutical past by those who work in the profession.

2. Relating to the public: It seems equally important that the public become aware of the historic and aesthetic values of artifacts and

equipment of bygone days used in the practice of the healing arts. If meaningfully presented, pharmaceutical and medical exhibits can be an important means of entertaining and educating the public.

3. Relating to state historical societies, and national and state museums and art galleries: One often finds many individuals zealous in community matters within their immediate locale who are at the same time indifferent about similar concerns at the state or national level. At the other extreme, as is the case in many countries in the Old World, national museums, galleries, and monuments that ornament the capitals and large cities attract all of the attention to the neglect of historical sites and centers in rural areas or small towns. Each should have its fair share of attention. State, provincial, and national institutions in the United States and Canada can improve and expand the quality and quantity of their cultural services. With rich and varied depositories and exhibitions, as well as adequate manpower and resources, museum directors, curators, and specialists can reconstruct, update, and maintain historical exhibits of lasting value for entertaining and educating larger audiences.

In the pharmacy museums and collections that are described in this publication, the viewer can discern in a most concrete way the special kinds of services and skills offered by the profession, and its development and progress through the years. Thus one comes to understand and appreciate in a unique way the long tradition and excellent performance of a humanistic calling to which we are all grateful.

Notes

1. Edward Kremers—a pioneer American educator and historian of pharmacy—gave a noteworthy report on this restoration in *The Badger Pharmacist,* No. 2 (April 1930), pp. 1–13. This unique collection, which was so beautifully displayed in the State Historical Society of Wisconsin at Madison, continued to entertain and inspire visitors for over half a century. It was, however, dismantled several years ago. It is hoped that it will be revived at a future date.

2. Several pharmaceutical collections are still awaiting installation for public viewing, some of which were previously on exhibit. Mention can be made of the early Chicago Drug Store at the Chicago Historical Society and the Old Time Apothecary Shop at The Lederle Laboratories Division of The American Cyanamid Company at Pearl River, New York. Others were dismantled, such as the Little Pharmacy in Virginia; The Charles Feke's Apothecary Shop Window in Rhode Island; and The Billingsley's Ye Old Apothecary Shop in Texas.

3. See S. Hamarneh, *Temples of the Muses and a History of Pharmacy Museums,* (Tokyo: The Naito Foundation, 1972), pp. 59–73.

4. Ibid., and S. Hamarneh, *Origins of Pharmacy and Therapy in the Near East,* (Tokyo: The Naito Foundation, 1973), pp. 1–23.

Bibliographic Guide

This is a concise, selected, and partly annotated bibliography intended as a brief list or introductory guide to the literature. It covers topics related to museology and to the history of pharmacy, its tools, and related arts and antiques. It may be useful to museum staff members, antique collectors, and researchers in the history of the healing arts, especially pharmacy, and the tools and equipment used in and related to them. Entries and categories are not comprehensive but will provide helpful references on means of identifying, evaluating, preserving, and displaying such artifacts and furnishings.

Under each of the following topics and categories, entries are listed in alphabetical order by authors or by titles of periodicals.

Periodicals on Museums and Museology

American Collector: A monthly published by the Crain Consumer Group, 740 Rush Street, Chicago, Illinois 60611. Started in 1970.

American Heritage: A bimonthly, published by the American Heritage Publishing Co., 10 Rockefeller Plaza, New York, New York 10020. Started in 1950. The American Heritage Society is also the publisher of the bimonthly *Americana.*

Antique Collector: A monthly, published in England, Oakfield House, Perrymound Road, Haywards Heath, Sussex RH16 3DH, England; in the United States, P.O. Box 10103, Des Moines, Iowa 50340.

Antique Monthly: "the nation's fine antiques newspaper") P.O. Box 2274, Birmingham, Alabama 35201. Published since 1968.

The Antiques Journal: A monthly (formerly *The American Antiques Journal* incorporating *Western Collector*) published by the Babka Publishing Co., Box 1046, Dubuque, Iowa 52001. It began publication in January 1946 and features important articles.

Apollo: "The Magazine of Arts," Denys Sutton, editor. Published in England, 22 Davis Street, London, WIS 1LH, England; in the United States, 75 Rockefeller Plaza, New York, New York 10019. Published since 1872.

Art News: Ten issues a year, P.O. Box 969, Farmingdale, New York 11737. Founded in 1902.

Beiträge Zur Geschichte der Pharmazie: A quarterly published by the International Society for the History of Pharmacy, Beilage der *Deutchen Apotheker-Zeitung* since 1949, illustrated. An important periodical, especially for Germanic pharmacy. Likewise see *Pharmaziegeschichtliche Rundschau,* Beiläge zur *Pharmazeutischen Zeitung.*

The Burlington Magazine: A bimonthly publication of Burlington Publications Ltd., Elm House, 10–16 Elm Street, London WC1, England.

Canadian Antiques Collector: A bimonthly, suite 406, 200 St. Clair Avenue West, Toronto, M4V 929, Ontario; M.F. Goldenberg, publisher. It started in 1966 with interest in "the rare and beautiful" and the motto "without a knowledge of and feeling for the past we cannot build as we should in the present and for the future."

The Connoisseur: Eight issues per year. It was founded in 1901, acquired by William R. Hearst in 1927, and is published by The National Magazine Co. Ltd. England, Vauxhall Bridge Road, London, SW4 1HF, England; in the United States, Olney Road and Mowbray Arch, Norfolk, Virginia 23510. William Allan, editor.

Craft Horizons: A bimonthly publication of the American Crafts Council, 44 West 53d Street, New York, New York 10019. Started in 1941.

Curator: A quarterly publication of the American Museum of Natural History, Central Park West at 79th Street, New York, New York 10024. Started in 1958 with useful articles, views, and opinions related to museology.

Early American Life: A bimonthly official magazine of the Early American Society Inc., P.O. Box 1831, Harrisburg, Pennsylvania 17105. Publishing began in 1970 to "advance understanding of American social history and modern interpretations of early arts, crafts, furnishings, and architecture."

Hobbies: A monthly "magazine for collectors" published by the Lightner Publishing Corporation, 1006 South Michigan Avenue, Chicago, Illinois 60605, since 1896.

The Magazine Antiques: A monthly for collectors and amateurs by Straight Enterprises Inc., 551 Fifth Avenue, New York, New York 10017; Wendell Garrett, editor and publisher. This magazine is a leading periodical in the field and has been issued since 1922. A commulative index of volumes 1–40 appeared in New York City, 1941. Alice Winchester et al., edited *The Antique Book,* containing illustrated articles from the first 56 volumes (1922–1949) (New York: Wyn, 1950), 319 pages; *Collector and Collections, the Antiques Anniversary Book* (New York, 1961), 165 pages, with illustrations and portraits (some in color).

The Museologist: A quarterly for the museum profession and an official publication of northeast conference museums; 657 East Avenue, Rochester, New York 14607. Started in 1942.

Museum: A quarterly review, successor to *Mouseion,* published by UNESCO, 7 Place de Fontenoy, 75700 Paris, France, Anne Erdös, editor. It started in 1949 and emphasizes activities and means of research in the field of museology.

Museum News: A bimonthly published as the journal of the American Association of Museums, 1055 Thomas Jefferson Street, N.W., Washington, D.C. 20007, since January 1924. The association also issues the *AAM Bulletin* for general news and classified advertisements related to museology.

Museums Journal: A quarterly published by the Museums Association, 87 Charlotte Street, London, WIP 2BX, England. Started in July 1901. It superseded the Association's *Report of Proceedings* published 1890–1900. The association also publishes, since 1961, the monthly bulletin, *Museums Association,* which carries museum news and related notices.

Old Stuff: A bimonthly ("about old times everybody loves") published by Windermere Communications Inc., 148 E. Lancaster Avenue, Wayne, Pennsylvania, 19087. Started in 1971.

Pharmacy in History: A quarterly published by the American Institute of the History of Pharmacy, University of Wisconsin, Madison, Wisconsin 53706. An indispensable periodical for anyone interested in pharmacy's past and artifacts. Started in 1959.

Smithsonian: A monthly published by the Smithsonian Associates, 900 Jefferson Drive, Washington, D.C. 20560. It covers a wide range of topics from popular science and museology to American culture and ecology. Started in 1970.

Spinning Wheel: Published ten times a year by the American Antiques and Crafts Society, Fame Avenue, Hanover, Pennsylvania 17331. Started in 1945.

Historical and Bibliographical References

Andersen, D., *Antique Furniture from Danish Prescription Pharmacies* (Copenhagen, 1948), 416-page edition of 1944 *Gammelt Dansk Apoteksinventar* with English introduction and captions of various pharmaceutical antiques mainly preserved in the Copenhagen Medical–Historical Museum and the Aarhus Museum; well illustrated.

Bender, George, and John Parascandola (editors), *Historical Hobbies for the Pharmacist* (Madison, Wisconsin, 1974). American Institute of the History of Pharmacy's 1973 symposium includes articles on pharmaceutical antiques (M.R. Harris); glassware (J.K. Crellin); philately (G.B. Griffenhagen); ephemera (W.H. Helfand); books (C. Reitman); and archeology (J.L. Grimm). Reprinted (with amendments) 1980.

DaCosta, Beverly (editor), *Historic Houses of America* (New York, American Heritage Publications Co., 1971). A guidebook with an introduction by Marshall B. Davidson.

Drake, T.G.H., "Antiques of Interest to the Apothecary," *J. Hist. Med.,* 15(1960): 31–44. Includes English delftware jars and pill tiles, mortars, medicine spoons, medicine chests, pill boxes, pap boats, posset pots, and infant feeding bottles and warmers.

Griffenhagen, George B., and L.B. Romaine, "Early U.S. Pharmaceutical Catalogues," *Amer. J. Pharm.,* 131(1959): 14–33. Convenient guide to drug and equipment catalogs in the United States. Useful in dating and tracing evolution of pharmaceutical pieces.

Guitard, E.H., *Manuel d'Histoire de la Littérature Pharmaceutique,* (Paris: Caffin, 1942), 138 pp. Contains pharmaceutical bibliography in alphabetical order with biographies of authors.

Häfliger, J.A., *Pharmazeutische Altertumskunde* (Basel, 1931). Well-documented source of information on pharmaceutical containers and equipment.

Hamarneh, Sami, "Early Arabic Pharmaceutical Instruments," *J. Amer. Pharm. Assoc., Pract., Pharm. Ed.,* 21(1960): 90–92 (tablet molds and strainers); "Arabic Glass Seals on Early 8th-Century Containers for materia medica,"

Pharmacy in History, 18(1976): 95–102; "Excavated Surgical Instruments," *Annali dell'Instituto e Museo di Storia della Scienze,* 2(1977): 3–14; *Pharmacy Museums USA* (Madison, Wisconsin, 1972), 1st edition, with useful bibliography; and *Temples of the Muses and a History of Pharmacy Museums* (Tokyo, 1972), especially useful with respect to Middle Eastern–Japanese artifacts, but also contains many illustrations of Occidental equipment, containers, and interiors.

Matthews, Leslie G., *Antiques of the Pharmacy* (London: G. Bell, 1971). Wide coverage by types of material, viz., pottery, metal, glass, wood; also drug chests, proprietary medicines, and printed materials. Bibliography and list of principal collections of pharmaceutical artifacts in Britain and the United States; and *The Royal Apothecaries* (London: Wellcome Historical Medical Library, 1967), xiv + 191 pp., with 13 plates, illustrations. An important work on the history of British pharmacy.

Schmitz, Rudolf, *Mörser Kolben und Phiolen, aus der Welt der Pharmazie,* (Stuttgart: Franckh'sche Verlagshandlung, 1966); 208 pp. A historical survey of pharmacy with numerous illustrations.

Schneider, Wolfgang, *Grundfragen der Pharmazie-Geschichte* (Stuttgart, 1959), in *Veröffentlichungen d. Intern. Gesellsch. f. Gesch. d. Pharm.,* n.s., vol. 1.

Somlo, Jean and Thomas, *Pharmaceutical Antiques and Collectables with Price Guide* (Manchester, Vermont: Forward Color Productions, 1970). A price guide of United States pharmaceutical antiques with 17 full-color plates.

Sonnedecker, Glenn, *Kremers and Urdang's History of Pharmacy,* 4th edition (Philadelphia: J.B. Lippincott, 1976); indispensable work, especially on American Pharmacy, with footnotes and appendixes. It contains an "International list of pharmacy museums" compiled by George B. Griffenhagen, pp. 396–417. See also G. Sonnedecker et al., *Some Bibliographic Aids for Historical Writers in Pharmacy,* (Madison, Wisconsin: American Institute of the History of Pharmacy, 1958); and "Some Pharmaco-historical guidelines to the Literature," *Am. Jr. Pharm. Ed.,* 23(1959), 143–172.

Trease, George Edward, *Pharmacy In History* (London: Balliere, Tindall and Cox, 1964), vii + 265 pp.; especially British pharmacy, with illustrations.

Urdang, G., and F.W. Nitardy, *Squibb Ancient Pharmacy* (New York: 1940). Intended as a catalog of the famed collection now part of the Smithsonian collections, the book with its many illustrations and detailed descriptions is a valuable guide to pharmaceutical glass, ceramics, and wooden containers, as well as mortars and pestles; mostly pre-nineteenth century European artifacts.

Winchester, Alice, *How to Know American Antiques* (New York, Dodd, Mead & Co., 1953).

Pictorial History of Pharmacy

Boussel, Gerald, *Histoire Illustrée de la pharmacie* (Paris: Guy le Plat, 1949).

Carson, Gerald, *One for a Man, Two for a Horse* (Garden City, New York: Doubleday, 1961), 128 pp., with illustrations of patent medicines.

Griffenhagen, G.B., *Medicine Tax Stamps Worldwide* (Milwaukee, Wisconsin: American Topical Association, 1971); see also his "Philatetic War on Drug

Abuse," *Drug Forum,* 3 (Fall, 1973), 1–36; and, with J.H. Young, "Old English Patent Medicines in America," paper 10, *United States National Museum Bulletin 218* (Washington D.C.: Smithsonian Institution, 1959), pp. 155–183.

Hamarneh, Sami, "Drawings and Pharmacy in Al-Zahrāwī's Surgical Treatise," paper 22, *United States National Museum Bulletin 228* (Washington, D.C.: Smithsonian Institution, 1961), 81–94; also "At the Smithsonian . . . Exhibits on Pharmaceutical Dosage Forms," *Jour. Amer. Pharm. Assoc.,* n.s., 2(1962): 478–479; and "Pharmacy in Prints," *ibid.* 10(1970): 216–220.

Hechtlinger, Adelaide, *The Great Patent Medicine Era, or without benefit of doctor* (New York: Madison Square Press, 1970). Beautifully illustrated; on patent medicines and folklore.

Hein, Wolfgang Hagen, *Die pharmacie in der Karikatur* (Frankfurt am Main: Goviverlag, 1964), 222 pp., with illustrations and text in English and German.

Helfand, William H., *Drugs and Pharmacy in Prints* (Madison, Wisconsin: American Institute of the History of Pharmacy, 1967), 53 pp., with illustrations reproduced from the author's personal collection; also his "Medicine and Pharmacy in French Political Prints," *Trans. and Stud. Coll. of Phys. of Philadelphia,* 4th ser., vol. 42, no. 1(July 1974), pp. 14–33; and *Medicine and Pharmacy in American Political Prints (1765-1870)* (Madison, Wisconsin: American Institute of the History of Pharmacy, 1979).

Hollander, Eugen, *Die Karikatur und Satire in der Medizin,* 2d edition, (Stuttgart, F. Enke, 1921), 404 pp., with illustrations (some in color).

Holzmair, Eduard, *Medicina Nummis* (Vienna: D.J. Weiner, 1937); containing description of Joseph Brettauer's Collections, covering the entire field of medals and numismatics in medicine, pharmacy, and allied sciences with 25 plates and over 250 illustrations.

Kisch, Bruno, "Collecting Medical Coins and Medals," *Ciba Symposia* 9(1948): 793–824.

MacKinney, Loren, and Thomas Herndon, *Medical Illustrations in Medieval Manuscripts* (Berkeley–Los Angeles: University of California Press, 1965), 263 pp., in two parts: (1) Early medicine in illuminated manuscripts; (2) medical miniatures in extant manuscripts with a checklist. It contains illustrations and plates, some in color, on all areas of the healing arts including pharmacy.

Pedrazzini, Carlo, *La Farmacia Sorica ed Artistica Italiana,* (Milan: Ed. Vittoria di Guido Ciarrocca, 1934), 592 pp. with important historical illustrations.

Peters, Hermann, *Der Arzt und die Heilkunst in der Deutschen Vergangenheit* (Leipzig: E. Diederichs, 1900), 136 pp., with 153 illustrations covering the period from the fifteenth century through the eighteenth; one of the earliest of its kind on the history of pharmacy.

Phillpotts, Eden, *A Museum Piece* (London–New York: Hutchinson, 1943), 264 pp., with illustrations.

Sonnedecker, Glenn, and S.A. Ives, *Pharmacy Through Four Centuries,* (Madison, Wisconsin: 1957), 29 pp; guide to an exhibit commemorating the seventy-fifth anniversary of the University of Wisconsin's School of Pharmacy; see also Sonnedecker's *Evolution of Pharmacy*, 1965, 19 pp., reprinted under the auspices of the American Institute of the History of Pharmacy in the 13th edition of *Remington Pharmaceutical Sciences*, (Easton, Pennsylvania: Mack Publishing Co., 1965), pp. 10–28.

Storer, Horatio R., *Medica in Nummis;* Malcolm Storer, editor, (Boston: Wright and Potter, 1931). Contains a detailed descriptive list of coins, medals, and jetons in the health field including pharmacy. Entries in subdivisions are arranged in alphabetical order.

Wallis, Henry, *Italian Ceramic Art* (London: B. Quaritch, 1904), xxix + 177 pp.; particularly on early Renaissance Majolica, with color illustrations. See also his other important works by the same publisher: *Oakleaf Jars*, 1903, xli + 92 pp. (on fifteenth-century Italian wares showing Moorish influence in a limited edition of 250 copies with illustrations in color); *The Art of the Precursors*, 1901, xxii + 99 pp. (on early Italian majolica with 25 color plates and other illustrations); and *Italian Ceramic Art, Figure Design and Other Forms of Ornamentation in the 15th-Century Italian Majolica,* 1905.

Wittop, Koning, D.A., *Art and Pharmacy*, 4 vols. (Deventer, The Netherlands: The Ysel Press, 1957–1976). An important work, beautifully illustrated with accurately identified reproductions in color and captions in four modern languages. The illustrations appeared earlier in the Dutch pharmaceutical calendars.

Zekert, Otto, *Kunst in Medizin und Pharmazie* (Vienna, 1956), 90 pp., plus 40 plates. A yearbook of the "Heilmittelwerke" series, with indexes of names and places mentioned.

Zigrosser, Carl, *Ars Medica* (Philadelphia: Philadelphia Museum of Arts, 1959 printing), 91 pp., containing a collection of medical prints presented to the museum by Smith Kline and French Laboratories.

Collectors Guidebooks

Bradford, Ernie D.S., *Antique Collecting* (London: English Universities Press, 1963), 215 pp. A "teach yourself" manual for collectors with illustrations.

Burcaw, G. Ellis, *Introduction to Museum Work* (Nashville, Tennessee: American Association for State and Local History, 1975), 202 pp.

Butler, Joseph T., *American Antiques (1800–1900)* (New York: Odyssey Press, 1965), 203 pp. A historical collector's guide with illustrations and color plates.

Callahan, Clair Wallis (pseud. Ann Kilborne Cole), *Antiques: How to Identify, Buy, Sell, Refinish, and Care for Them* (New York: McKay, 1957), 246 pp., including bibliography. Illustrations by Cynthia Rockmore.

Cowi, Donald, and Keith Henshaw, *Antique Collector's Dictionary*, (London: Arco Publications, 1962), 208 pp., with illustrations and plates.

Doane, Ethel Mary, *Antiques Dictionary* (Brockton, Massachusetts: 1949), viii + 290 pp., with bibliography and illustrations.

Eberlein, Harold Donaldson, and Abbot McClure, *The Practical Book of American Antiques*, rev. ed. (Garden City, New York: Halcyon House, 1948), iv + 390 pp. Contains 257 illustrations and drawings and deals with artifacts, industries, trade history, and collecting.

Greene, Edward Lee, *Landmarks of Botanical History* (Washington D.C.: Smithsonian Institution, publ. no. 1870, 1909). A study of certain epochs of botanical science, part. 1, prior to A.D. 1562.

Hamarneh, S. "Coinage in Islam," *The Islamic Quarterly,* no. 3–4, vol. 5(1960): 99–101; "For The Collector, Facts and Artifacts," *Pharmacy History,* 6(1961): 48–50; "Dental Exhibition and Reference Collection at the Smithsonian," *Health Services Report,* 87(1972): 291–303.

Hayword, Helen, editor, *The Connoisseur's Handbook of Antique Collecting* (London: The Connoisseur, 1960), 320 pp., with an introduction by L.G.G. Ramsey. A dictionary of furniture, silvers, ceramics, glass, fine art objects, industries, and trade.

Hughes, George Bernard, *The Antique Collector's Pocket Book,* 1st American edition (New York: Hawthorn Books, 1965), 351 pp. (1st edition in London, 1963, under the title *The Country Life Collector's Pocket Book);* illustrations by Therle Hughes.

Kendrick, Grace, *The Antique Bottle Collectors,* rev. ed. (Sparks, Nevada: Western Printing and Publishing Company, 1964) 3d edition, 1966, 92 pp.; explains and identifies old American medicinal bottles and glasswares for collectors, with illustrations by Laura Mills.

McClinton, Katherine (Morrison), *Antique Collecting* (Greenwich, Connecticut: Fawcett Publications, Inc., 1952), 144 pp., illustrated; abridged from *Antique Collecting for Everyone.* See also her *Collecting American Victorian Antiques* (New York: Charles Scribner's Sons: 1966), 288 pp., with illustrations and bibliography.

Philip, D.A., *Antiques Today* (London: Miller, 1960), 157 pp.; mainly on furniture and pottery.

Rush, Richard H., *Antiques as an Investment* (Englewood Cliffs, New Jersey: Prentice-Hall, 1968), 536 pp., with illustrations and drawings by Julia Rush.

Savage, L. George, *The Antique Collector's Handbook* (London, Barrie and Rockliff, 1959), 304 pp., including bibliography, with illustrations and drawings by Frederick Curl.

Vivian, Margaret Cordelia, *Antique Collecting* (London: Pitman, 1937), xvi + 234 pp., with illustrations and plates.

Way, Reginald Philip, *Antique Dealer* (London: M. Joseph, 1956), 211 pp. (1st American edition, New York: MacMillan, 1956), includes autobiography.

Yates, Raymond Francis, *The Antique Collector's Manual* (New York, Harper, 1952), viii + 303 pp., contains detailed and wide-range data for the general collector.

Museums and Museology

Adam, Thomas Ritchie, *The Civic Value of Museums* (New York: American Association for Adult Education, 1937), xi + 114 pp. This is no. 4 of the association's series of publications on the significance of museums as educational centers. See also his *The Museum and Popular Culture* (same publisher, 1939), ix + 177 pp., devoted to studies in the social significance of adult education in the United States.

Babelon, Jean Pierre, *The Museums of France,* translated by James Brockway (New York: Meredith Press, 1968), 160 pp., with illustrations and plates.

Bazin, Germain, *The Museum Age,* translated from the French by Hane Van Buis Cahill, 1st American edition (New York: Universities Press, 1967), 307 pp. Contains history of collections, galleries, and museums, with illustrations.

Benoist, Luc, *Musée et Museologie* (Paris: Presses Universitaires de France, 1960), 126 pp., with illustrations and bibliography.

Burcow, G. Ellis, *Introduction To Museum Work* (Nashville, Tennessee: The American Association for State and Local History, 1975). The topics discussed include: history, definitions, organization; support, care, and security of museums and collections; evaluation of exhibits, visitors, educational activities, and architecture; and preservation, public image, theories, and practical applications relative to museums and society.

Coleman, Laurence Vail, *Historic House Museums* (Washington, D.C.: American Association of Museums, 1933), xii + 187 pp., illustrated with plates, a map, and a directory. See also his *The Museum in America,* 3 vols., by the same publisher, 1939. Coleman also wrote on university and small company museums and historical buildings.

Gerstner, Patsy A., *The Care and Exhibition of Medical History Museum Objects* (Cleveland, Ohio: The Cleveland Health Sciences Library, 1974), mimeographed, 47 pp.

González, Ramón Jordi, *Propaganda y Medicamentos, Anetecedentes Históricos de un Fraude a la Sociedad* (Barcelona: Edición Continental, 1977), 99 pp., with illustrations.

Griffenhagen, George B., *Pharmacy Museums* (Madison, Wisconsin: American Institute of the History of Pharmacy, 1956), revised under the title: "International List of Pharmacy Museums," with references in G. Sonnedecker's, *Kremers and Urdang's History of Pharmacy,* 4th ed. (Philadelphia: Lippincott, 1976), pp. 396–417.

Guldbeck, P.E., *The Care of Historical Collections* (Nashville, Tennessee: American Association for State and Local History, 1972).

Hall, Edward T. *The Hidden Dimension* (Garden City, New York: Doubleday, and Company, 1966).

Hamarneh, Sami, "History of the Division of Medical Sciences," paper 43, *United States National Museum Bulletin* 240, Washington, D.C.: Smithsonian Institution, pp. 269–300. See also his "Smithsonian Exhibits on Pharmaceutical History," *Journal Amer. Pharm. Ass.,* n.s., 5(1965): 434–435 and 438; and "The Pharmacy Museum at Krakow," *Amer. Jour. Hosp. Pharm.,* 21(1964): 266–273.

Hamarneh, S., *Temples of the Muses and a History of Pharmacy Museums* (Tokyo: The Naito Foundation, 1972), x + 146 pp., with illustrations, some in color, and describing museums in the Old and New Worlds.

Harrison, Holly, *Changing Museums, Their Use and Misuse* (London: Longmans, 1967), x + 110 pp., with illustrations, 8 plates, and bibliography. It emphasizes educational aspects.

Holmes, Martin R., *Personalia* (London: Museums Association, 1957), 23 pp., intended as a manual for museum personnel and techniques.

Hudson, Kenneth, *A Social History of Museums, What the Visitors Thought* (Atlantic Highlands, New Jersey: Humanities Press, 1975), 210 pp.

Kalz, Herbert and Marjorie, *Museum, U.S.A., A History and a Guide* (Garden City, New York: Doubleday, 1965), x + 395 pp. See also the authors' *Museum Adventures* (New York: Coward-McCann, 1969), 253 pp., discussing discoveries and exhibits of 47 museums in the United States, especially those geared toward science and technology.

Knorr, Heinz Arno, *Handbuch der Museen und Wissenschaften Sammlungen in der D.D.R.* (Halle-Saale: Fachstelle für Heimatmuseen beim Ministerium für Kultur, 1963), xv + 520 pp., with illustrations and map.

Larrabee, Eric, *Museums and Education* (Washington, D.C.: Smithsonian Institution Press, 1968).

Low, Theodore L., *The Museum as a Social Instrument* (New York: The Metropolitan Museum of Art, 1942), 70 pp.

Markham, Sydney Frank (compiler), *Directory of Museums and Art Galleries in The British Isles* (London: Museums Association, 1948), 302 pp., with illustrations.

Prakash, Satya, *Museums and Society* (Baroda, India: University of Baroda, Department of Museology, 1964), 59 pp.

Ripley, Dillon, *The Sacred Grove* (New York: Simon and Schuster, 1969), 159 pp. Contains essays and lectures on museums and their role in education and the transmission of cultures. It is one of the finest texts of its kind providing meaningful and profound information on museums' contributions to human knowledge and creativity.

Schwartz, Alvin, *Museums, The Story of America's Treasure Houses,* (New York: Dutton, 1967), 256 pp., with illustrations, portraits, a map, and bibliography.

Taylor, Francis Henry, *Babel's Tower, The Dilemma of the Modern Museum* (New York: Columbia University Press, 1945), containing useful and delightful discussions.

Taylor, Frank A. *Research in Exhibits* (Washington, D.C.: Smithsonian Institution Press, 1968).

Wittlin, Alma Stephanie, *The Museum, Its History and Its Task in Education* (London: Routledge and Kegan Paul, 1949). A fascinating discussion on the history and place of museums in education, updated by the author's useful enlargement upon this theme in his *Museums, in Search of a Useful Future* (Cambridge, Massachusetts: Massachusetts Institute of Technology Press), 1970.

Tools and Equipment of the Apothecary's Art

Including balances and weights, mortars and pestles, microscopes, pill tiles and machines, drug mills and containers, suppository molds, percolators, show globes, and other equipment.

Berriman, Algernon Edward, *Historical Metrology* (New York: Dutton, 1953).

Blair, A., "On Drug Mills," *Proc. American Pharm. Association*, 23 (1875): 575–587.

Bradbury, Savile, *The Evolution of the Microscope* (Oxford–New York: Pergamon, 1967), x + 357 pp. An important work with bibliography and illustrations.

Cazala, Roger, M.A., *Les Mortiers d'Apothicaires* (Grenoble, France: Imp. Allier, 1953), 108 pp., in paperback.

Child, Ernest, *The Tools of the Chemist, Their Ancestry and American Evolution* (New York: Reinhold, 1940), 220 pp. Useful for the history of balances, glass and porcelain wares, ovens, and filters.

Clay, Reginald S., and Thomas H. Court, *The History of the Microscope* (London: Griffin, 1932), 266 pp. A useful compilation from original documents and the study of original specimens from the beginning up to the introduction of the achromatic microscope; with illustrations.

Couch, J.F., "The Early History of Percolation," *American Journal of Pharmacy*, 91(1919): 16–25.

Crellin, John K., *Medical Ceramics in the Wellcome Institute of the History of Medicine* (London: Wellcome Institute, 1969), vii + 304 pp. Describes about 2,500 ceramic pieces of British and Dutch origins related to pharmacy and the healing arts in three parts: (1) Drug jars, pots, pill tiles, mortars, and tin-glazed and stone ware; (2) nursing devices and hygenic utensils including pap boats, food warmers, spittoons, and urinals; (3) medical devices and inhalers, and surgical bleeding bowls.

Crellin, J.K., and D.A. Hutton, "Comminution and English Bell-Metal Mortars, c. 1300–1850," *Medical History*, 17(1973): 266–287.

Crellin, J.K., and J.R. Scott, "Drug weighing in Britain, c. 1700–1900," *Medical History*, 13(1969): 51–67; also *Glass and British Pharmacy, 1600–1900* (London: Wellcome Institute, 1972).

DaSilva, Marbins, *A Evolução do Almofariz Peninsular de Séc. XIII–XIX* (Lisbon: Academia Nacional de Belas Artes, 1975), 11 pp. text and captions, and 33 figures.

Dorveaux, P., *Les Pots de Pharmacie* (Toulouse, France, 1923).

Drake, T.G.H., "Antique English Delft Pottery of Medical Interest," *Canadian Medical Association Journal*, 39(1938): 585–88.

Folch, G., *Catalogo de Morteros de Farmacia* (Madrid, 1966).

Griffenhagen, G.B., *Tools of the Apothecary* (Washington, D.C.: American Pharmaceutical Association, 1957), 30 pp., reprinted from a series appearing in 1956, *J. Amer. Pharm. Assoc., Pract. Pharm. Ed.*, with monographs on the mortar and pestle, pharmaceutical balances, pharmaceutical weights, suppository molds, pill tiles and spatulas, pill machines, filtration equipment, drug percolators, the drug mill, lozenges, capsules, and tablets. See also his, "The Mysterious Origin of the Show Globe . . . A Symbol of Pharmacy," *Rx Health*, October 1964, pp. 26–31; "The Evolution of the Medicine Chest," *The Antiques Dealer*, 26(October and November 1974), pp. 32–35 and 37–39 respectively; "Mortars and Pestles," ibid, 25(October and November 1973), pp. 28–31, and 30–32, 62–63 respectively; "The Apothecary Jar, An Historical Sketch," *The Science Counselor*, 22(June 1959), pp.

41–44, 68–69; "The Pharmacy in History," *The Jour. of the International Col. of Surgeons,* 29(1958): 788–803; "Poison Bottles and Safety Closures," *J. Amer. Pharm. Assn.,* n.s., 1(1961): 563–66; and "The World's Fanciest Pill Bottles," *Today's Health,* 42(December 1964), pp. 42–46 and 69–70.

Griffenhagen, G.B., and Ernst W. Stieb, *Tools of the Apothecary, A Select Bibliography* (Madison, Wisconsin: American Institute of the History of Pharmacy, 1975), 13 pp., mimeographed.

Hagelstein, Robert, *The History of the Microscope* (New York, 1944).

Hamarneh, S., "Early Arabic Pharmaceutical Instruments," *Jour. Amer. Pharm. Assn.,* 21(1960): 90–92; also "The Pharmaceutical Exhibition at the Smithsonian," *Amer. Jour. of Hospital Pharmacy,* 23(1966): 605–9; "The Pharmaceutical Collection at the Smithsonian," *Pharmacy History,* 9(1967): 55–64; "The First Recorded Appeal for the Unification of Weight and Measure Standards in Arabic Medicine," *Physis,* 5(1963): 230–248; "At the Smithsonian . . . Exhibits on Pharmaceutical Dosage Forms," *Jr. Amer. Pharm. Assn.,* 2(1962): 478–79; "Medicine U.S.A. . . . Damascus International Fair," ibid., 5(1965): 28–29; "Smithsonian Exhibits on Pharmaceutical History," ibid., pp. 434–35 and 438; and "Excavated surgical instruments from Old Cairo, Egypt, *Annali Dell'Instituto e Museo di Storia della Scienza di Firenze,* 2(1977): 3–14.

Howard, G.E., *Early English Drug Jars* (London, 1931).

Janot, M.M., *Les Capsules medicamenteuses* (Paris, 1944).

Kisch, Bruno, *Scales and Weights, A Historical Outline* (New Haven: Yale University Press, 1965), xxi + 297 pp.

Kohlhaussen, H., et al., *Alte Apothekengefässe* (Biberach an der Riss: Thomae, 1960).

LaWall, Charles H., *Four Thousands Years of Pharmacy* (Garden City, N.Y.: Garden City Publishing Co., Inc., 1927); and "An Interesting Collection of Mortars," *Jr. Amer. Pharm. Assoc.,* 23(1934): 570–581.

Lloyd, J.T., "Development of the Pharmaceutical Mortar," *Pract. Druggist,* 52(January 1934), pp. 12–17.

Lothian, Agnes, "Some English Bell Founders and Their Mortars," *Chemist and Druggist,* 169(1958): 704–711; also "Bird Designs on English Drug Jars," ibid., 161(1954): 672–77; "English Leeches and Leech Jars," ibid., 172(1959); 152–4, 157–8; "The Pipe-Smoking Man on 17th Century English Drug Jars," ibid., 163(1955): 566–68; "Saints on Drug Jars," ibid., 159(1953): 598–603; and "Two Centuries of Dated Drug Jars," ibid., 177(1962): 722–25.

Machabey, Armand, *La Métrologie dan Les Musèes de Province* (Paris: Centre Nationale de la Recherche Scientifique, 1961), 512 pp. On the history of weights and measures in France since the thirteenth century with description of museum collections; also *Mémoire sur l'histoire de la balance et de la balancerie* (Paris, 1949).

Matthews, Leslie G. "Apothecary Pill Tiles," *Transactions of the English Ceramic Circle,* 7(1970), part 3, pp. 200–209, giving systematic description of manufacturing, design, color, and dates of about 110 tiles.

Miles, George C., *Contribution to Arabic Metrology* (New York: American Numismatic Society, 1958), including description of early Arabic glass weights with illustrations.

Milliken, W.M., "Majolica Drug Jars," *Bull. Med. Library Assoc.*, 32(1944): 293–303.

Planten, H.R., *The Art of Capsulating* (New York, 1909).

Rackham, B., *Catalogue of Italian Majolica* (London: Victoria and Albert Museum, 1940); also *Italian Majolica* (same publisher, 1st edition, 1952; 2d edition, 1963).

Rupko, Roland E., *A Dictionary of English Weights and Measures*, (Madison, Wisconsin: University of Wisconsin, 1968), xvi + 224 pp., tracing the historical development of Anglo-Saxon weights up to the nineteenth century.

Segers, E.G., *Faiences Pharmaceutiques Anciennes* (Brussels, 1969).

Skinner, Frederick G., *Weights and Measures; Their Ancient Origins and their Development in Great Britain* (London: H.M.S.O., 1967), xii + 117 pp. A science museum survey with illustrations, 16 plates, map, and tables.

Snyder, G., *Wägen und Waagen* (Ingelheim am Rhein, Germany: C.H. Boehringer Sohn, 1957).

Thomann, H.E., *Die delfste Pootenkämer der J.R. Geigy A.A. Basel* (Ruschlikon, Switzerland, 1964).

Urdang, George, and F.W. Nitardy, *The Squibb Ancient Pharmacy*, (New York: E.R. Squibb, 1940), 190 pp. Contains identification, description, and illustrations of the E.R. Squibb and Sons Collection brought from Germany in 1932. It was displayed in Chicago and New York, and donated to the American Pharmaceutical Association in Washington, D.C. The association deposited the collection for permanent exhibition at the Smithsonian Institution's National Museum of History and Technology (renamed the National Museum of American History in 1980). See pages 26-27.

Wilson, Bill, and Betty, *19th Century Medicine in Glass* (Amador City, California: 19th Century Hobby and Pub. Co., 1971).

Wittop Koning, Dirk A., *Delft Drug Jars* (Deventer, The Netherlands: Bock-en Steen drukkerij "De Ijsel," 1954). Also his *Nederlandse Vijzels* (Deventer: Davo, 1953), 114 pp., with summaries in English and French. A monumental work on Dutch mortars, their decorative motifs, and their makers and illustrations. See also his (with K.M.C. Zevenboom) *Nederlandse Gewichten*, (Leiden: Rijkmuseum, V.d. Gesch. d. Naturwetensch, 1953), 264 pp. on Dutch weights, their marks and makers with illustrations and plates.

Wood, J.R. *Tablet Manufacture, Its History, Pharmacy and Practice* (Philadelphia, 1906).

Woodbury, Roberts, *History of the Grinding Machine* (Cambridge, Massachusetts: Massachusetts Institute of Technology, 1959), 191 pp. An authoritative text on the subject, with illustrations.

Ceramics, Majolica, Faience, and Delft Ware

Brigitte, Klesse, *Majolica* (Cologne: Bachem, 1966), with introduction by Erich Kollmann. A reliable text, covers Persian, Syrian, Turkish and European pottery and its development; numerous illustrations.

Castiglioni, Arturo, "Apothecary Jars in Antiquity, Renaissance and in the American Colonies," *Ciba Symposia*, 6(1945), pp. 2045–85; very general, with illustrations.

Changler, Maurice H., *Ceramics in the Modern World* (Garden City, New York: Doubleday, 1967), 192 pp. Emphasizes man's first technological coming-of-age with illustrations and bibliography.

Chompert, Joseph, *Les Faiences françaises primitives d'après les apothicaireries hospitalières* (Paris, n.d. [1940s]), with preface by H. Haug. See also his useful work, *Reportoire de la majolique Italienne*, 2 vols. (Paris, 1949).

Conradi, Helmut Peter, *Apothekenglässer im Wandel der Zeit* (Würzburg: Jal verlag, 1973), 199 pp. with 118 illustrations and 10 graphic tables. This is volume 10 of the series *Quellen und Studien zur Geschichte der Pharmazie*, Rudolf Schmitz (Marburg), editor.

DaSilva, A.C. Correia et al., *Exposição de faianças Portuguesas de Farmácia* (Lisbon: Biblioteca Nacional de Lisbon, 1972), 100 pp. plus 36 plates.

DeJonge, Caroline H., *Delft Ceramic* (New York: Praeger, 1970), including those ceramics of Italian, English, and Dutch origins.

Drey, Rudolf E.A., *Apothecary Jars: Pharmaceutical Pottery and Porcelain in Europe and the East 1150–1850* (London and Boston: Faber and Faber, 1978); with a glossary of terms used in apothecary jar inscriptions.

Fisher, Stanley W., *English Ceramics* (London, 1966), including discussions of earthen and stone wares, delft, and cream wares as well as porcelain.

Fourest, Henry-Pierre, *Les Faiences de Delft* (Paris: Presses Universitaires de France, 1957); discusses forms, techniques, decor, ornamentations, and styles in general with illustrations.

Frothingham, Alice W., *Talavera Pottery* (New York: Hispanic Society of America, 1944); describes the society's fine and important collection with illustrations.

Giacomotti, Jeanne, *La Majolique de la Renaissance* (Paris: Presses Universitaires de France, 1961). An authoritative and illustrated text that covers sixteenth-century technique, style, decor, and marks, and their diffusion into European craftsmanship, as well as imitations and restoration. It contains also a bibliography and graphic charts. In addition, the author wrote several texts on ceramics and their development in Europe up to the nineteenth century, such as his two volume work, *La Céramique* (Paris: Flammarions, 1934); with illustrations and plates in color.

Godden, Geoffry A., *Illustrated Encyclopaedia of British Pottery and Porcelain* (London: Jenkins, 1966), xxvi + 390 pp.; adequately illustrated.

Hein, W.-H. and D.A. Wittop Koning, *Deutsche Apotheken-Fayencen* (Frankfurt am Main: Govi-Verlag, 1977), 160 pp., being the fifth in the series of *Monographen zur Pharmazeutischen Kulturgeschichte;* a guide to German tin-glazed and delft wares.

Hillier, Bevis, *Pottery and Porcelain (1700–1914)* (London: Weidenfeld and Nicolson, 1968); including social history of the decorative arts on pottery and Wedgwood in Europe and North America.

Honey, William Bowyer, *European Ceramic Art*, 2 vols. (London: Faber, 1949–1952); including its development from the end of the Middle Ages to about 1815, with plates, maps, and a bibliography.

Howard, Geoffrey E. *Early English Drug Jars* (London: The Medici Society, 1931), 3 + 49 pp., with plates in color. It discusses posset pots, pill tiles, and barbers bowls as well; includes a glossary compiled by Charles J.S. Thompson.

Hudig, Ferrand Whaley, *Delften Fayence* (Berlin: Schmidt, 1929).

Kingery, William Davis, *Introduction to Ceramics* (New York: Wiley, 1960), 781 pp., with illustrations.

Klein, Adelbert et al., *Islamische Keramik* (Berlin and Düsseldorf: Hetjens-Museum, 1973); illustrated. Describes pottery exhibitions.

Lewis, G., *A Picture History of English Pottery* (London, 1956).

Liverani, Giuseppe, *Five Centuries of Italian Majolica* (New York: McGraw-Hill Book Company, Inc., 1960), 260 pp., with illustrations and plates in color.

Lothian, A., "Dutch drug jars and their marks," *The Alchemist*, 16(1952): 216–221; and "Vessels for Apothecaries, English Delft Drug Jars," *The Connoisseur Year Book* (London, 1953), pp. 113–121.

Miller, J. Jefferson, II, *English Yellow-Glazed Earthenware* (Washington, D.C.: Smithsonian Institution Press, 1974); discusses forms, decorative techniques, and modes of manufacturing.

Quimby, Ian M.G., editor, *Ceramics in America: Winterthurl Conference Report* (Charlottesville: University Press of Virginia, 1973); including salt-glazed stone and pearl wares.

Rackham, Bernard, *Italian Maiolica* (London, Faber, 1952; 2d ed., 1963); discusses origins, techniques, and aesthetic considerations of types and centers of ceramic manufacturing with illustrations and plates. Also his authoritative work, *Catalogue of Italian Maiolica*, 2 vols. (London: Victoria and Albert Museum, 1940), with illustrations and plates.

Ray, Anthony, *English Delftware Pottery in the Robert Hall Warren Collection, Ashmolean Museum* (Oxford-London: Faber, 1968), with preface by Nigel Warren. Includes tin-glazing and Lambeth and Bristol delft.

Savage, George, *English Pottery and Porcelain* (London, 1961), 43 pp. (American edition, New York, Universe Books); *Eighteenth-Century German Porcelain* (London: Rockliff, 1958), 242 pp., foreword by H. Weinberg, also illustrated; and *Porcelain Through the Ages* (London: Penguin Books, Ltd., (2d ed.), 1961).

Towner, D.C., *English Cream-Coloured Earthenware* (London, 1957).

Wakefield, H., *Victorian Pottery* (London, 1962).

Walker, H., "Ancient Pharmacy Jars," *The Connoisseur*, 20(1908): 251–254.

Wittop Koning, D.A., *De oude Apotheek* (Delft, 1966).

Porcelain, Wedgwood, Glassware, and Medicinal Bottles

Inevitably there are overlaps in the entries when a work covers more than one subject or type of artifact.

Amaya, Mario, *Tiffany Glass* (London: Studio Vista, 1966), 168 pp. Louis Comfort Tiffany (1848–1933), a chemist, painter, and interior designer, introduced the new metallic iridescent glass for opalescent window shows and improved interior decoration. He designed the "favrite" handmade blown glass in a variety of colors and shapes as decorative accessories, borrowing from Islamic and Oriental designs. This is a survey of the art that has been associated with the Tiffany name since the 1880s; with illustrations and plates in colors.

Barber, Edwin Atlee, *American Glassware, Old and New* (Philadelphia, Patterson and White, 1900), 112 pp., with a sketch on the early glass industry in the United States and a guide for collectors of antique bottles. See also his *The Pottery and Porcelain of the U.S.*, 2d edition, (New York: Putnam, 1901), 539 pp., with illustrations.

Bates, Virginia T., and Beverly Chamberlain, *Antique Bottle Finds in New England* (Peterborough, New Hampshire: Noone House, 1968), 80 pp., with illustrations.

Belknap, Eugene McCamly, *Milk Glass* (New York: Crown, 1949), 327 pp.; a useful illustrated reference with introduction by George S. McKearin.

Bemrose, G., *Nineteenth-Century English Pottery and Porcelain* (London, 1952).

Buten, Harry M., *Wedgwood Counterpoint* (Merion, Pennsylvania: Buten Museum of Wedgwood, 1962).

Charleston, Robert Jesse (editor), *English Porcelain (1745–1850)* (London: E. Benn, 1965), 183 pp.; also *World Ceramic, an Illustrated History* (London: Hamlyn, 1968), 352 pp., with illustrations, maps, and bibliography.

Cox, Warren Earle, *The Book of Pottery and Porcelain*, 2 vols. (New York: Crown, 1944), with 3,000 illustrations laid out by A.M. Lounsbery, maps and colored plates (2d edition in 2 vols., London, 1970). It broadly discusses European tin-glazed wares, pottery, and porcelain in the Old and New Worlds.

Daniel, Dorothy, *Cut and Engraved Glass, 1771–1865* (New York: M. Burrows, 1950), 441 pp. A collector's guide to American glassware with drawings by Sigismund Widberg.

Davis, Marvin, *Antique Bottles* (Medford, Oregon: Gandee Printing Center, 1967), 62 pp.; illustrations and colored plates by Terry Skibby.

Dorveaux, Paul, *Les pots de pharmacie*, 2d ed. (Toulouse, France: 1923), 86 pp. and 13 plates, covering the history of drug jars with glossary for identification of inscriptions.

Godden, Geoffrey, A., *Caughley and Worcester Porcelain, 1775–1800* (New York: Praeger, 1969), xxi + 166 pp. (British ed., London: Jenkins); and *The Handbook of British Pottery and Porcelain Marks* (same publisher, 1968), 197 pp.

Haggar, Reginold George, *Concise Encyclopaedia of Continental Pottery and*

Porcelain (London, 1960); and *Glass and Glass Makers* (New York: Roy Publishers, 1962), 80 pp., with illustrations.

Hannover, Emil, *Pottery and Porcelain* (London: E. Benn, 1925). English translation by Bernard Rackham. A comprehensive and authoritative handbook for collectors and historians covering the history of ceramics, porcelain, and stoneware in Europe and the Near East, with illustrations, maps, indexes, and a bibliography.

Haynes, E. Barrington, *Glass Through the Ages,* rev. ed. (London: Penguin Books, Ltd., 1959), 309 pp.; an historical, illustrated survey.

Honey, W.B., *German Porcelain* (London, Faber, 1947), xv + 56 pp., 2d edition, 1954; *English Pottery and Porcelain* (London: Blac, 1933), xvi + 270 pp., 5th edition, 1964; *French Porcelain of the 18th Century* (London: Faber and Faber, 1950), xv + 78 pp.; *Old English Porcelain* (same publisher), 202 pp. (2d ed., 1948); and *Wedgwood Ware* (same publisher), 1948, xv + 35 pp., plus plates and bibliography.

Hudig, F.W., *European Glass* (Boston: Houghton Mifflin Co., 1926), xxxvi + 96 pp., including a history of glassmaking and decorations.

Hughes, G. Bernard, *Victorian Pottery and Porcelain* (London: Country Life, 1959), 184 pp., and *English Glass for the Collector* (same publisher), 1958, an illustrated manual.

Knittle, Rhea Mansfield, *Early American Glass* (London: Appleton-Century, 1937; New York, 1939), xxiii + 496 pp.

Lee, Ruth Webb, *Early American Pressed Glass* (Farmington Center, Massachusetts, 1933); *Victorian Glass* (Northborough, Massachusetts, 1944), describing a variety of types; and *Sandwich Glass* (same publisher, 1947), an illustrated history of glass manufacturing at Boston and Sandwich, Massachusetts.

McKearin, Helen, and George S., *Two Hundred Years of American Blown Glass* (Garden City, N.Y.: Doubleday, 1950) complements an earlier work entitled, *American Glass* (New York: Crown, c. 1950). It contains illustrations, drawings, and plates by James L. McGreery.

Metz, Alice Hulet, *Early American Pattern Glass* (Westfield, New York: Guide Publishing Co., 1958), 243 pp., describing about 1,500 patterns, uses, and terminology.

Pesce, Giovanni, *Maioliche Liguri da Farmacia presentazione del Prof. Giorgio del Guerra* (Milan: Edizioni Luigi Alfieri, 1960).

Phillips, Helen T., *Antique Bottles* (Cheyenne, Wyoming: Logan, 1967), including history and description of the author's collection.

Thorn, C. Jordan, *Handbook of Old Pottery and Porcelain Marks* (New York: Tudor, 1947), with foreword by John M. Graham.

Thorpe, W. A., *English Glass* (London: Black, 1935).

Van Rensselaer, Stephen, *Early American Bottles and Flasks,* 3d edition by Edmund Edwards, (Stratford, Connecticut: J.E. Edwards, 1969), with introduction by Charles B. Gardner.

Watson, Richard, *Bitters Bottles and Supplement,* 2 vols. (New York–Camden, New Jersey: T. Nelson and Sons, 1965–1968), with illustrated listings of bottles according to shapes, labels, advertising, and manufacturing.

Antique Fakes, Restoration, and Conservation

Feller, R.L., "Control of the Deteriorating Effects of Light upon Museum Objects," *Museum,* vol. 17, 1964.

Gairola, T.R., *Handbook of Chemical Conservation of Museum Objects,* (Department of Museology, University of Baroda, India, 1960), xi + 101 pp.

International Institute of Conservation, *London Conference on Museum Climatology,* International Institute of Conservation, 6 Buckingham Street, London WC2N 6BA, England, 1967.

Kingery, W.D. (editor), *Ceramic Fabrication Processes,* Cambridge, Massachusetts: Massachusetts Institute of Technology Press, 1958, xi + 253 pp., with illustrations and diagrams.

Kurz, Otto, *Fakes* (New York: Dover, 1967).

Lee, Ruth Webb, *Antique Fakes and Reproductions* (Farmington, Massachusetts, 1938), 224 pp.; rev. ed., enlarged (Northboro, Massachusetts: Lee, 1950), xviii + 317 pp.

Lewis, Ralph, *Manual for Museums* (Washington, D.C.: National Park Service, 1976).

Lucas, Alfred, *Antiques, Their Restoration and Preservation,* 2d edition, rev. (London: Arnold, 1932), 240 pp. (first edition, 1924).

Mendax, Fritz, *Art, Fakes and Forgeries* (London, 1955).

Organ, Robert M., *Design for Scientific Conservation of Antiquities* (London: Butterworth and Company, 1968), xi + 497 pp.

Plenderleith, Harold James, *The Conservation of Antiquities and Works of Art* (London: Butterworth and Company and Oxford University Press, 1962). The first edition, under the title *The Preservation of Antiquities,* was published in London, by the Museums Association, 1934, viii + 71 pp. and includes a bibliography.

Plenderleith, H.J., and Werner, A.E., *The Conservation of Antiquities and Works of Art* (London: Oxford University Press, 1968).

Savage, George L., *Forgeries, Fakes and Reproductions* (London: Barrie and Rockliff, 1963), xiii + 312 pp., bibliography, an illustrated handbook for the collector; and *The Art and Antique Restorer's Handbook* (New York: Philosophical Library, 1954), 140 pp., a dictionary of material and processes used in the restoration and preservation of all kinds of works of art.

Texas Historical Commission, *Thoughts on Museum Conservation* (Austin, Texas: Texas Historical Foundation, 1976).

Thomson, Gary, *The Museum Environment* (London: Butterworth and Company, 1978).

Yates, Raymond Francis, *Antique Fakes and Their Detection* (New York: Harper, 1950), x + 229 pp., with photographs and drawings by the author.